D1444082

To Improve Health and Health Care

Volume VIII

Stephen L. Isaacs and
James R. Knickman, Editors

Foreword by Risa Lavizzo-Mourey

~m~ To Improve Health and Health Care

Volume VIII

The Robert Wood Johnson
Foundation Anthology

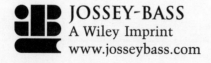

JOSSEY-BASS
A Wiley Imprint
www.josseybass.com

Published by Jossey-Bass
A Wiley Imprint
989 Market Street, San Francisco, CA 94103-1741   www.josseybass.com

Jossey-Bass books and products are available through most bookstores. To contact Jossey-Bass directly call our Customer Care Department within the U.S. at (800) 956-7739, outside the U.S. at (317) 572-3986 or fax (317) 572-4002.

Jossey-Bass also publishes its books in a variety of electronic formats. Some content that appears in print may not be available in electronic books.

ISSN: 1547-3570
ISBN: 0-7879-7635-0

Printed in the United States of America
FIRST EDITION
PB Printing   10 9 8 7 6 5 4 3 2 1

–ɯ–Table of Contents

Foreword   ix
Risa Lavizzo-Mourey

Editors' Introduction   xi
Stephen L. Isaacs and James R. Knickman

Acknowledgments   xvii

The Editors   xix

The Contributors   xxi

Section One: National Programs   1

1   **Taking on Tobacco: The Robert Wood Johnson
Foundation's Assault on Smoking**   3
James Bornemeier

2   **The SmokeLess States Program**   29
Karen K. Gerlach and Michelle A. Larkin

3   **Reducing Youth Drinking: The "A Matter of Degree"
and "Reducing Underage Drinking Through
Coalitions" Programs**   47
Susan G. Parker

4   **The Robert Wood Johnson Foundation's
Commitment to Nursing**   73
Carolyn Newbergh

5   **The Turning Point Initiative**   99
Paul Brodeur

Section Two: A Closer Look   125

6   The Chicago Project for Violence Prevention   127
    Digby Diehl

Section Three: Inside The Robert Wood Johnson Foundation   153

7   The Robert Wood Johnson Foundation:
    The Early Years   155
    Joel R. Gardner and Andrew R. Harrison

8   National Programs: Understanding The Robert Wood
    Johnson Foundation's Approach to Grantmaking   177
    Robert G. Hughes

    Index   199

    Table of Contents, To Improve Health
    and Health Care 1997   207

    Table of Contents, To Improve Health
    and Health Care 1998–1999   208

    Table of Contents, To Improve Health
    and Health Care 2000   209

    Table of Contents, To Improve Health
    and Health Care 2001   210

    Table of Contents, To Improve Health
    and Health Care Volume V   211

    Table of Contents, To Improve Health
    and Health Care Volume VI   212

    Table of Contents, To Improve Health
    and Health Care Volume VII   213

–ⵡ–Foreword

Even if the scandals that have rocked corporate America had not reached the world of philanthropy and Congress were not considering restrictive legislation, it would still be imperative for foundations to report openly, honestly, and comprehensively to their boards and to the public. By law, foundations are accountable to their boards of trustees—and, of course, to regulatory agencies, principally the Internal Revenue Service, and state attorneys general. But in a larger sense, foundations are public trusts, serving as stewards of private resources for the public good. As such, they have an obligation to be publicly accountable.

Accountability can be viewed in at least two ways. It can refer to financial accountability—being transparent and ethical in keeping the books and reporting on financial transactions. IRS Form 990-PFs are publicly available and accessible to all. This is a major step toward promoting financial accountability, even if, like most tax forms, the 990-PF is an arcane and not always easily understood document.

The second type of accountability—programmatic accountability—receives much less attention. It refers to transparency in letting the public know what a foundation has done with the private dollars it has been given or bequeathed, why it did so, and, under the best of circumstances, what lessons can be learned from its grantmaking.

I am fortunate to be leading a foundation that has such a strong tradition of public accountability, of both the financial and the programmatic varieties. Since its earliest days, the Foundation's presidents have used the *Annual Report* to share information and concerns about substantive health matters. Our newsletter, *Advances,* provides an even broader public with capsule descriptions of the Foundation's grants and the activities of our grantees. Reports of more than 1,500 grants are now posted on The Robert Wood Johnson Foundation Web site, as are findings from Foundation-funded research.

In addition, the Foundation produces *To Improve Health and Health Care: The Robert Wood Johnson Foundation Anthology,* a book series published annually by Jossey-Bass. At the convergence of evaluation, communications, and program analysis, *The Robert Wood Johnson Foundation Anthology* series opens up our programmatic books to the public. Volumes produced over the past eight years contain chapters ranging from large topics, such as the Foundation's efforts to reduce smoking and to improve care toward the end of life, to small projects, such as New Mexico's Recovery High School and San Francisco's Homeless Prenatal Program. By critically examining the work of its grantees and revealing the inner workings of the Foundation itself, *The Robert Wood Johnson Foundation Anthology* also helps to demystify the often opaque world of philanthropy.

Through these mechanisms, The Robert Wood Johnson Foundation seeks to achieve programmatic, as well as fiscal, accountability, and to meet our obligations as a public trust. We may not have gotten it quite right yet, but we are pointed in the right direction.

Princeton, New Jersey   Risa Lavizzo-Mourey
September 2004   President and CEO
                                            The Robert Wood Johnson Foundation

–ɯ–Editors' Introduction

With assets of approximately $8 billion, The Robert Wood Johnson Foundation is the nation's fifth-largest foundation. To carry out its simple but daunting mission of improving the health and health care of all Americans, the Foundation strives to foster innovation, develop ideas, disseminate information, and enable a wide range of committed people to devote their energies to improving the nation's health and well-being. While the Foundation's primary mechanism for effecting change in health and health care systems, practice, and policy is its awarding of approximately $400 million of grants each year, the Foundation also energizes the health field by convening experts, by creating synergy among its grantees and partners, and by disseminating knowledge about key issues in health and health care through its Web site, the Web sites of key grantees, and a range of publications produced by its staff in Princeton and by its grantees.

The Robert Wood Johnson Foundation is committed to a set of principles that guide both its grantmaking and its internal operations. It focuses on improving the health and health care of the most vulnerable individuals in our society; it is inclusive and nonpartisan in its strategies; it addresses significant and challenging problems and continues working on them long enough to have an impact; and it values the passion, commitment, and energy of both its grantees and its staff.

The Foundation structures it staff and grantmaking activities around four portfolios:

- One portfolio targets eight objectives, each addressing a major health issue facing our nation. Four of the objectives relate to health care (for example, improving the quality of medical care and expanding health insurance coverage). The other four relate to health and disease prevention (for example, reducing childhood obesity and strengthening the public health system).

- A second portfolio seeks to develop human capital, that is, to strengthen the health workforce.

- A third portfolio supports direct services (and the testing of new ideas that will improve services) to vulnerable populations, such as those living in inner cities or rural areas, or people suffering from chronic illness.

- A fourth portfolio looks for innovative, pioneering ideas that don't fall within traditional categories.

The initial five chapters in this year's *Robert Wood Johnson Foundation Anthology* look at the Foundation's national programs aimed at improving health.

- Chapter One, by James Bornemeier, provides an overall examination of the Foundation's work in tobacco control. The Foundation entered the field in the early 1990s and pursued what, in retrospect, appears as a comprehensive strategy to reduce smoking.
- Chapter Two, by Karen Gerlach and Michelle Larkin, chronicles the SmokeLess States program, which supported statewide tobacco-control coalitions throughout the nation. The authors provide an insiders' view of how SmokeLess States evolved from a program using a number of educational and policy tools to one focused exclusively on advocacy to change state-level tobacco policies.
- Chapter Three, by Susan Parker, looks at another broad topic aimed at changing unhealthy behavior—in this case, drinking among underage youth and binge drinking. It discusses the Foundation's two key alcohol-abuse prevention initiatives: A Matter of Degree, which seeks to curb excessive drinking by building coalitions of colleges and their surrounding communities, and Reducing Underage Drinking Through Coalitions, which encourages partnerships to discourage drinking among high school students.

■ Chapter Four, by Carolyn Newbergh, reviews the Foundation's investments to strengthen the nursing profession. Although the Foundation has sporadically entered and exited from specific programs over the years, it has demonstrated a commitment to nursing since its inception as a national philanthropy in 1972.

■ Chapter Five, by Paul Brodeur, analyzes Turning Point, the Foundation's most significant initiative to strengthen public health. This initiative, funded jointly by The Robert Wood Johnson Foundation and the W.K. Kellogg Foundation, has supported public-private partnerships at state and local levels since 1996.

Every year, the *Anthology* features one chapter putting a small local program under the microscope. This is one way to give a human face to the Foundation's activities and to illustrate that not all of its grantmaking involves large programs designed to affect nationwide change in policy or practice.

■ In Chapter Six, Digby Diehl examines the Chicago Project for Violence Prevention, which is attempting to reduce gun violence in some of that city's highest-crime neighborhoods.

One goal of the *Anthology* is to demystify the world of philanthropy, at least insofar as philanthropy is practiced by The Robert Wood Johnson Foundation. This year's *Anthology* contains two chapters that illuminate the Foundation from the inside.

■ Chapter Seven, written by Joel Gardner and Andrew Harrison, tells the story of the Foundation's early days. It begins with the establishment of a small, local New Jersey foundation established in 1936 by Robert Wood Johnson, the president of Johnson & Johnson; explores the challenges faced when it became a national philanthropy in 1972; and concludes in 1975, when the large new national Foundation had three years of experience under its belt.

■ Chapter Eight, by Robert Hughes, provides an insider's view of the Foundation's principal mechanism for managing its grants—its national programs. This structure, which relies on outside organizations and experts to administer programs, emerged in the early 1970s as a way to balance the tension between maintaining a small staff of Foundation program officers and exercising tight oversight of grantees.

As is obvious from this summary, this year's *Robert Wood Johnson Foundation Anthology* covers a wide range of initiatives to improve health and health care. If there is a common thread running through the chapters—at least a significant number of them, including those on nursing, tobacco control, and the end of life—it is the importance of knowing when to leave a program or a field, how to exit gracefully, and how and whether to sustain the work after the Foundation's support has ended.

In the past, little thought had to be given to exit strategies and sustaining programs. This was, perhaps, because government could be expected to pick up the financing of successful programs, or because there was an expectation on the part of both grantees and Foundation staff that The Robert Wood Johnson Foundation's support would continue indefinitely. So the focus in the past was on the replication of successful models and taking projects "to scale" so that government—preferably federal—would notice and ultimately support them. Moreover, in the generally good economic times that characterized much of the 1980s and 1990s, the Foundation's resources kept growing. New programs were authorized, but many old programs continued. The Foundation began a large number of initiatives that did not have a natural endpoint, and it made open-ended commitments to grantees. Both new and perpetual challenges could, it seemed, be addressed simultaneously.

Changing times force new patterns of thinking. The economy is no longer growing as it did in the previous decades. The federal government has devolved the financing of social programs to states and localities; it is no longer expected to absorb even successful initiatives begun with foundation support. After a long period dedicated to examining its priorities, The Robert Wood Johnson Foundation made the decision to leave a number of fields, even as it is making long-term commitments to others.

All of these factors have led to a reconsideration of how long to continue funding programs and how to exit from them. As former Foundation president and chief executive officer, Steven Schroeder, quoting from the Kenny Rogers song, wrote, "You've got to know when to hold 'em; know when to fold 'em." The Robert Wood Johnson Foundation does not have the answer (nor does anybody else) to the question of how long to stay with programs. What the Foundation has learned, however, is that a few years is probably not long enough to influence the development of a field or to bring about social change, and that it is necessary to think about sustainability from the earliest stages of program development. It has convened a staff task force, called "roots and wings," to consider how best to leave programs and fields; is assisting some grantees in sustaining their efforts; and remains committed to finding ways to continue work begun with Foundation support that remains essential.

San Francisco Stephen L. Isaacs
Princeton, New Jersey James R. Knickman
September 2004 Editors

~ⅢⅢ~Acknowledgments

The Robert Wood Johnson Foundation *Anthology* series is a collaborative effort, and we owe a debt of gratitude to the many people who have worked with us in the editing and production of Volume VIII. Within The Robert Wood Johnson Foundation, David Morse, especially, has been an invaluable partner. An active participant from beginning to end, he has brought thoughtfulness, sound judgment, and creativity to the project. In addition to writing the foreword, Risa Lavizzo-Mourey reviewed all the chapters and made valuable suggestions for their improvement. Ayorkor Gaba did an outstanding job of pulling together materials and helping us in a variety of other ways, as did her successor, Katherine Muessig. Molly McKaughan's editorial review of the chapters led to improvement in all of them. Deborah Malloy, Nancy Giordano, Sara Wilkinson, and Sherry De Marchi made it possible for communications between San Francisco and Princeton to flow smoothly. Paul Moran, Tim Crowley, Carol Owle, Mary Castria, Carolyn Scholer, Ellen Coyote, and Russ Henshaw handled financial transactions with their usual efficiency. Hope Woodhead oversaw distribution matters impeccably, and Barbara Sherwood made sure the book was always displayed in the Foundation's lobby and got to the right people outside of the Foundation. Richard Toth and Lydia Ryba checked the accuracy of the dollar amounts and dates of all Foundation grants mentioned in the book. Hinda Feige Greenberg, Katherine Flatley, and Mary Beth Kren were of great help in identifying and finding material needed by editors and authors alike.

Beyond the Foundation, C. P. Crow again demonstrated why he is considered a legendary editor. Carolyn Shea continued to be an extraordinary fact checker. Lauren MacIntyre converted hand-marked edited copy into printed text with amazing speed and accuracy. At Health Policy Associates, Elizabeth Dawson was a trusted colleague in all aspects of editing and producing the *Anthology,* and Greta McKinney performed her bookkeeping duties conscientiously, as usual.

A number of people reviewed individual chapters, and we wish to acknowledge their contribution. The reviewers included Bobbie Berkowitz, Carol Chang, Susan Hassmiller, James Ingram, Nancy Kaufman, Janet Malcolm, Dwayne Proctor, Pamela Russo, Steven Schroeder, Pauline Seitz, Gary Slutkin, and Victoria Weisfeld.

Finally, we wish to pay special thanks to the *Anthology's* outside review committee: Susan Dentzer, Frank Karel, William Morrill, Patti Patrizi, and Jonathan Showstack. Their insightful comments have been critical in maintaining the fair and balanced analysis and the high quality of the writing that has characterized the *Anthology* series since 1997.

S.L.I. and J.R.K.

–ɯ–The Editors

Stephen L. Isaacs, J.D., is a partner in Isaacs/Jellinek, a San Francisco–based consulting firm, and president of Health Policy Associates, Inc. A former professor of public health at Columbia University and founding director of its Development Law and Policy Program, he has written extensively for professional and popular audiences. His book *The Consumer's Legal Guide to Today's Health Care* was reviewed as "the single best guide to the health care system in print today." His articles have been widely syndicated and have appeared in law reviews and health policy journals. He also provides technical assistance internationally on health law, civil society, and social policy. A graduate of Brown University and Columbia Law School, Isaacs served as vice president of International Planned Parenthood's Western Hemisphere Region, practiced health law, and spent four years in Thailand as a program officer for the U.S. Agency for International Development.

James R. Knickman, Ph.D., is vice president for research and evaluation at The Robert Wood Johnson Foundation. He oversees a range of grants and national programs supporting research and policy analysis to better understand forces that can improve health status and delivery of health care. In addition, he is in charge of developing formal evaluations of national programs supported by the Foundation. During the 1999–2000 academic year, he held a Regents' Lectureship at the University of California, Berkeley. Previously, Knickman was on the faculty of the Robert Wagner Graduate School of Public Service at New York University. At NYU, he was the founding director of a university-wide research center focused on urban health care. His publications include research on a range of health care topics, with particular emphasis on issues related to financing and delivering long-term care. He has served on numerous health-related advisory committees at the state and local levels and spent a year working at New York City's Office of Management and Budget. Currently, he chairs the board of trustees of Robert Wood Johnson University Hospital in New Brunswick. He completed his undergraduate work at Fordham University and received his doctorate in public policy analysis from the University of Pennsylvania.

–ɯ–The Contributors

James Bornemeier is a writer with twenty-five years' experience in journalism as an editor and correspondent at the *Los Angeles Times, Philadelphia Inquirer,* and *Providence Journal.* He is now a New York City–based writing and editing consultant, working primarily with major charitable organizations such as the Ford Foundation, where he is a contributing editor of the *Ford Foundation Report,* The Robert Wood Johnson Foundation, the Goldman Sachs Foundation, and the New York Community Trust. From 1997 to 2003, he worked as public affairs officer at The Pew Charitable Trusts where he oversaw communications for the Culture and Public Policy programs. He is a graduate of Northwestern University.

Paul Brodeur was a staff writer at *The New Yorker* for nearly forty years. During that time, he alerted the nation to the public health hazard posed by asbestos, to depletion of the ozone layer by chlorofluorocarbons, and to the harmful effects of microwave radiation and power-frequency electromagnetic fields. His work has been acknowledged with a National Magazine Award and the Journalism Award of the American Association for the Advancement of Science. The United Nations Environment Program has named him to its Global 500 Roll of Honour for outstanding environmental achievements.

Digby Diehl is a writer, literary collaborator, and television, print, and Internet journalist. Recently honored with the Jack Smith Award from the Friends of the Pasadena Public Library, his book credits include *Angel on My Shoulder,* the autobiography of singer Natalie Cole; *The Million Dollar Mermaid,* the autobiography of MGM star Esther Williams; *Tales from the Crypt,* the history of the popular comic book, movie, and television series; and *A Spy for All Seasons,* the autobiography of former CIA officer Duane Clarridge. For eleven years, Diehl was the literary correspondent for ABC-TV's *Good Morning America* and was recently the book editor for the *Home Page* show on MSNBC. He continues to appear regularly on the morning news on KTLA. Previously the entertainment editor for KCBS television in Los Angeles, he was a writer for the Emmys and for the soap opera *Santa Barbara,* book editor of the Los Angeles *Herald Examiner,* editor-in-chief of art book publisher Harry N. Abrams, and the founding book editor of the *Los Angeles Times Book Review.* Diehl holds an M.A. in theater from UCLA and a B.A. in American studies from Rutgers University, where he was a Henry Rutgers Scholar. He is presently collaborating with Coretta Scott King on her memoirs.

Joel R. Gardner is a writer and oral historian who specializes in the history of private philanthropy. In that capacity, he has worked as a consultant to The Robert Wood Johnson Foundation since 1991. In addition, he has conducted oral history projects and written histories for The Pew Charitable Trusts and The John D. and Catherine T. MacArthur Foundation. He has written numerous articles for scholarly journals as well as general-interest publications. Most notably, his article "Oral History and Philanthropy: Private Foundations" appeared in *Journal of American History* in 1992. He has also written histories of Memorial Hospital of Burlington County, New Jersey, and the Tasty Baking Company, and conducted interviews on behalf of the Columbia University Oral History Research Office and the Getty Center for the Arts and Humanities. His interview for Columbia with Charles Scribner, Jr., became *In the Company of Writers,* published in 1991. He holds degrees in French, from Tulane University, and journalism, from UCLA, where he began his oral history career.

Karen K. Gerlach, Ph.D., M.P.H., is a senior program officer at The Robert Wood Johnson Foundation. She leads the Foundation's tobacco team and oversees programming in tobacco prevention and control. She is a member of the policy committee of the Society for Research on Nicotine and Tobacco and previously served on the section council for the

Alcohol, Tobacco, and Other Drugs Section of the American Public Health Association. She sits on the advisory committee for the state of Nebraska's tobacco control program. She completed her undergraduate work at Indiana University, her Ph.D. at the Indiana University School of Medicine, and her M.P.H. at Johns Hopkins University.

Andrew R. Harrison, Ph.D., received a B.A. in history from The George Washington University in 1988. He graduated Magna Cum Laude from that school and was admitted into its Phi Beta Kappa chapter. Following undergraduate school, Harrison attended Temple University where he received a Ph.D. in history. Currently, he works as the archivist for The Robert Wood Johnson Foundation and teaches as an adjunct professor at Philadelphia University and Community College of Philadelphia. He has taught more than 100 college courses in American, European, and World history, specializing in U.S. twentieth-century political and social topics. Harrison has published a book on the Philadelphia Soviet Jewry movement entitled *Passover Revisited* and has written a number of articles on Philadelphia's Jewish community.

Robert G. Hughes, Ph.D., is chief learning officer of The Robert Wood Johnson Foundation. His previous positions during fifteen years at the Foundation include director of program research and program vice president. His interests are in the areas of health policy research, philanthropy and social change, and organizational behavior. His responsibilities within the Foundation have included the Tobacco Policy Research and Evaluation Program, the Investigator Awards in Health Policy Research Program, the Substance Abuse Policy Research Program, and the Health Tracking Initiative. Between 1991 and 1994, he was the convener of the "substance abuse working group," the staff committee charged with developing and reviewing substance abuse programs. Hughes came to the Foundation from Arizona State University where he was an assistant professor in the School of Health Administration and Policy. He received his Ph.D. from the Department of Behavioral Sciences, Johns Hopkins School of Hygiene and Public Health, and was a Pew postdoctoral fellow at the University of California, San Francisco Institute for Health Policy Studies.

Michelle A. Larkin, R.N., M.S., is a senior program officer at The Robert Wood Johnson Foundation. Her work focuses primarily on tobacco-control policy, end of life, and improving the quality of care, including program development, design, and management. Prior to joining the Foundation, Larkin served as a health policy analyst at the Office on Smoking and Health at the Centers for Disease Control and Prevention in Washington, D.C. She was responsible for analyzing policy and legislative proposals related to state, national, and international tobacco prevention and control; coordinating and drafting the *Healthy People 2010* tobacco chapter; and working with the U.S. Domestic Policy Council on the Framework Convention on Tobacco Control. She also served as a legislative fellow for the United States Senate Labor and Human Resources Committee, working on tobacco control, poison control, managed care reform, and children's health issues. She has served on several federal review committees and workgroups. Larkin received her B.S. in nursing from the University of Pennsylvania, and worked as an oncology nurse for over a decade at the University of Maryland Medical System. After completing her M.S. in nursing/health policy from the University of Maryland, she was a Presidential Management Intern at the U.S. Department of Health and Human Services.

Risa Lavizzo-Mourey, M.D., M.B.A., is the fourth president and chief executive officer of The Robert Wood Johnson Foundation, a position she assumed in January 2003. She originally joined the staff in April 2001 as the senior vice president and director, health care group. Prior to coming to the Foundation, Lavizzo-Mourey was the Sylvan Eisman Professor of Medicine and Health Care Systems at the University of Pennsylvania, as well as director of the Institute on Aging. Lavizzo-Mourey was the deputy administrator of the Agency for Health Care Policy and Research, now known as the Agency for Health Care Research and Quality. While in government service, Lavizzo-Mourey worked on the White House Health Care Policy team, including the White House Task Force on Health Care Reform, where she cochaired the working group on quality of care. Lavizzo-Mourey has served on numerous federal advisory committees, and recently completed work as codirector of an Institute of Medicine study on racial disparities in health care that resulted in the publication of *Unequal Treatment, Confronting Racial and Ethnic Disparities in Health Care.* She is the author of numerous articles and several books. A member of the Institute of Medicine of the National Academy of Sciences, Lavizzo-Mourey earned her medical degree at Harvard Medical School followed by an M.B.A. at the University of Pennsylvania's Wharton School. After completing a residency in internal medicine at Brigham and Women's Hospital in Boston, Massachusetts, Lavizzo-Mourey was a Robert Wood Johnson Clinical Scholar at the University of Pennsylvania, where she also received her geriatrics training.

Carolyn Newbergh is a Northern California writer who has covered health care trends and policy issues for more than twenty years. Her freelance work has appeared in numerous print and online publications. As a reporter for *The Oakland Tribune,* she wrote articles on health care delivery for the poor as well as emergency room violence, AIDS, and the impact of crack cocaine on the children of addicts. She was also an investigative reporter for the *Tribune,* winning prestigious honors for a series on how consultants intentionally cover up earthquake hazards in California.

Susan G. Parker is a reporter with more than twenty years of experience, covering everything from police and courts to Congress to the war in Guatemala. She has written for *Time* magazine, the *Washington Post,* the *San Francisco Chronicle, USA Today, The Boston Globe,* and many other publications. As a foreign correspondent in Guatemala, she traveled to remote parts of the country to interview Guatemalans about the effects of war on their health, their beliefs about the emerging peace process, and their conversion to evangelical Christianity. She holds a master's degree from Harvard Divinity School and has had her own writing business since 1996, specializing in health, religion, and business topics. Her clients include The Robert Wood Johnson Foundation, Harvard University, Boston College, the U.S. Department of Justice, and Education Development Center, Inc. She is based in Cambridge, Massachusetts.

National Programs

1

Taking on Tobacco

The Robert Wood Johnson Foundation's Assault on Smoking

James Bornemeier

Editors' Introduction

The Robert Wood Johnson Foundation's tobacco-control grantmaking illustrates
the many tools available to a foundation committed to attacking a serious social
problem, and *The Robert Wood Johnson Foundation Anthology* series has featured half a dozen chapters that touch on a number of them.[1] In this chapter,
James Bornemeier, a freelance journalist specializing in philanthropy and health,
chronicles the entire panoply of Foundation programs to reduce smoking in the
United States.

    Although the Foundation's efforts appeared to be piecemeal, Borne-
meier observes that, in retrospect, one can make out a comprehensive grantmaking strategy. That strategy included, among other elements:

- Research to understand the most effective policy interventions, such as raising taxes on cigarettes, and to build a new field of tobacco-policy research

- Demonstration programs—for example, programs to test effective ways
  for people to stop smoking

- Advocacy aimed at counteracting the tobacco industry's influence on children (through the Center for Tobacco-Free Kids) and to effect policy change (through SmokeLess States coalitions)

- Development and dissemination of tobacco-cessation standards for managed care organizations

- Communications activities

The chapter offers a good case study of how a foundation can nurture a field by embracing all its aspects. It also provides insights about how foundations can work in areas where there is organized and powerful opposition. The tobacco industry certainly did not welcome the Foundation's efforts to reduce smoking. Indeed, the Foundation began its investments in tobacco control with some trepidation, and then only on the condition that programs be focused on reducing tobacco use by young people, for whom smoking was illegal. Even so, the tobacco industry raised legal challenges—all successfully met—to some of the Foundation's grantmaking approaches, particularly those which emphasized advocacy.

Bornemeier notes in his conclusion that the Foundation is in the process of reducing its involvement in the tobacco-control field and moving on to other priorities. This raises a final question—how will the field evolve without the support and encouragement the Foundation has given it over the past decade? The Foundation is keeping a watchful eye on developments.

---

1. Gutman, M., Altman, D. G., and Rabin, R. L., "Tobacco Policy Research." *To Improve Health and Health Care 1998–1999: The Robert Wood Johnson Foundation Anthology.* San Francisco: Jossey-Bass, 1999; Koppett, L., "The National Spit Tobacco Education Program." *To Improve Health and Health Care 1998–1999: The Robert Wood Johnson Foundation Anthology.* San Francisco: Jossey-Bass, 1999; Kaufman, N., and Feiden, K. L., "Linking Biomedical and Behavioral Research for Tobacco Use." *To Improve Health and Health Care 2000: The Robert Wood Johnson Foundation Anthology.* San Francisco: Jossey-Bass, 2000; Orleans, C. T. and Alper, J., "Helping Addicted Smokers Quit: The Foundation's Tobacco-Cessation Programs." *To Improve Health and Health Care, Vol. VI: The Robert Wood Johnson Foundation Anthology.* San Francisco: Jossey-Bass, 2003; Diehl, D., "The Center for Tobacco-Free Kids and the Tobacco-Settlement Negotiations." *To Improve Health and Health Care, Vol. VI: The Robert Wood Johnson Foundation Anthology.* San Francisco: Jossey-Bass, 2003; Chapter Two of this volume.

─ᴍ─ **F**or someone who can take considerable personal credit for the sustained battle against smoking over the past decade, Steven Schroeder offers remarkably little evidence to explain his motivation. "There was no flash of light," Schroeder recalled not long ago. "It was a combination of things. My training as an epidemiologist opened my eyes to the ravages of substance abuse, including tobacco. I had a couple of patients who died, and that really broke me up. One was a very nice African American woman in her late forties who had a congenital problem with her hip and finally got it replaced and was looking forward to a full life. But postoperative X-rays spotted a shadow on her lung, and she died soon after. I also remember a three-pack-a-day journalist, a really great guy. His wife called me at 6 A.M. one day. He had had a cardiac arrest. Both of my parents smoked—and quit, as did I. All these experiences had an effect on me."

Such experiences are woven into the fabric of millions of American lives. The scourge of substance abuse has strengthened, tested, and sundered families and posed enduring and largely intractable problems to society, but by most measures Schroeder's life had only been grazed by its perils and depredations. In 1990, in a timely happenstance for the researchers, advocates, scientists, attorneys, and activists who made up the vanguard of the tobacco-control community in this country, Schroeder was about to become the president of The Robert Wood Johnson Foundation. With the change of leadership came the de-facto mandate for Schroeder to step back and reevaluate the Foundation's mission. When he did, he saw an opportunity to get the Foundation involved in an area where it had had only a minimal presence. While he saw no flash of revelatory light, the opportunity did present itself as an obligation, and his decision changed the Foundation and helped transform the battlefield of tobacco control.

─ᴍ─ **A New Mission**

Before 1987, combating substance abuse was not even part of the Foundation's agenda. That year, substance abuse was included under the goal of reducing destructive behavior, one of ten Foundation priorities in the late 1980s. By 1997, substance abuse had become the single largest investment area, totaling more than a quarter of the Foundation's $900 million in grants and commitments.[1]

Schroeder arrived with more of a social-activist agenda than had previous presidents of the Foundation, and with the notion that the work of the Foundation should be "less about grantmaking areas and more about where the country should be."[2] At his first meeting with the board, as a candidate for president in November 1989, Schroeder made it clear that he wanted to make substance abuse, and within it tobacco control, the first among several proposed Foundation goals. The board was generally receptive, partly because the Foundation had done some work previously in the substance-abuse field, most visibly with the Partnership for a Drug-Free America, which it had begun supporting earlier in 1989 and which sought to deglamorize drugs, and Fighting Back, which began in 1989 and helped form community coalitions to reduce demand for alcohol and drugs.

At a February 1991 retreat, the board debated the wisdom of approving the substance-abuse goal, which, after considerable internal debate, had been refined to target "the irresponsible use of tobacco, alcohol, and drugs." To some trustees, taking on tobacco seemed a risky enterprise, given the staff's relative inexperience in the field. Others worried that the Foundation would be drawn into controversies over legalization and enforcement. With smoking already in decline, locking horns with the powerful tobacco industry struck some board members as problematic, if not wrongheaded. But the grim unavoidable statistics about tobacco's lethality was persuasive, and the board adopted the goal of "reducing the harmful effects and the irresponsible use of tobacco, alcohol, and drugs."[3] It insisted, however, that the Foundation's tobacco-control efforts focus initially on young smokers—for whom cigarettes were illegal. The first grant in the tobacco portfolio, $1.3 million to Stop Teenage Addiction to Tobacco, or STAT, was approved in 1991, and the Foundation's substance-abuse era had begun.

—◠◡◠— Americans and Tobacco

According the U.S. Centers for Disease Control and Prevention, or CDC, some 46 million adults in the United States smoke cigarettes—a behavior that will result in premature death or disability for half of all regular users.[4] Cigarette smoking is responsible for more than 440,000 deaths each year, or one in every five deaths. Paralleling this enormous health toll is the economic burden of tobacco use: smoking-related illnesses cost the nation more than $150 billion each year.

Because of shifts in pubic tolerance and various political, economic, and social influences, the use of tobacco has fluctuated significantly over the past century.[5] It increased dramatically between 1900 and the mid-1960s, rising during war years, dipping during the Great Depression. At its peak in 1963, annual consumption hit more than four thousand cigarettes per person age eighteen and up. The Surgeon General's report issued the following year linked smoking definitively to health problems and precipitated a general decline ever since, marked by occasional ups and downs. Tobacco use actually increased among young people between the early- and mid-1990s, as pro-use messages from the entertainment industry, mixed with ever more sophisticated marketing by the tobacco industry, along with other factors, had their effect. According to the University of Michigan's study, *Monitoring the Future,* the percentage of twelfth-graders who reported smoking during the previous month grew from 27.8 percent in 1992 to 36.5 percent in 1997. By 2002, the percentage had decreased to 26.7, and is expected to continue its downward trend. Despite the decreases, at least 4.5 million young people under the age of eighteen are current smokers.[6]

—⚏— A Start from Scratch

Once the board had adopted the substance-abuse goal in 1991, the Foundation's staff was faced with a steep learning curve. A new and controversial issue had been placed on the Foundation's agenda, and the lack of staff expertise was palpable. Robert Hughes, who is now the Foundation's chief learning officer, was asked by Schroeder to convene a substance-abuse working group. Hughes guided the twenty-odd member staff committee charged with developing the Foundation's new substance-abuse program, which included tobacco, alcohol, and illegal drugs.

"We were literally starting from scratch," Hughes recalled. "We had to get educated on the tobacco issue—who was doing what in the field—and deliberately set out to design programs that could play off the efforts of others." But relatively few philanthropic activities involving tobacco were under way, and those that did exist were on a remarkably small scale compared with the magnitude of the problem.

"We talked to experts and scientists and advocates to get the lay of the land," Hughes said. "The process was evolutionary in nature, and there was no master plan that we were working under. A large part of our agenda was assessing what kinds of resources were needed to get the field moving, because we wanted to get out of the box quickly." But, Hughes said, staff enthusiasm for the substance-abuse mission was tepid. "It was a tough sell," he recalled. "Most of the members of the working group did not choose to be in it." Two factors helped turn that attitude around. The early 1990s was a period of significant asset growth for the Foundation, so grant dollars for the new goal were not coming out of the budgets of existing programs. "Not having to compete for resources made our task much less controversial," Hughes said. More important, over time the Foundation's substance-abuse programs came to be seen as a kind of laboratory for fresh ways of doing things at the Foundation.

Since the early 1990s, The Robert Wood Johnson Foundation has funded nearly 522 grants out of its tobacco-control portfolio, ranging from $5,000, its smallest tobacco grant, to $99 million for SmokeLess States, its largest national program (see Table 1.1). The Foundation's approaches have been varied, encompassing research, policy interventions, prevention and cessation programs, education and advocacy, coalition building, leadership training, convening, and communications activities. The breadth of the tobacco-control strategy is suggested in such programs as Bridging the Gap, an interdisciplinary partnership of substance-abuse research experts working to improve the understanding of how policy and environmental factors affect alcohol, illicit drug, and tobacco use among young people; Smoke-Free Families, targeted at getting pregnant smokers to quit; Americans for Nonsmokers' Rights, focused on the dangers of secondhand smoke; and the National Spit Tobacco Education Program, organized to prevent people, especially young people, from taking up spit, or chewing, tobacco.[7]

The grants largely fall into four main strategic areas: policy research, state-based advocacy and coalition building, a national communications and strategy center, and cessation and treatment programs. "It wasn't apparent at first, but the tobacco portfolio became a very integrated effort," said Joe Marx, a senior communications officer at the Foundation, who has been on the tobacco-control team since the early 1990s. "Through regular conference calls and e-mail, each group knew what the others were doing. We had so many specialized resources that it was a case of 'what do we have, and how do we use it?' " While the Foundation may not have had a detailed vision in mind when it entered the tobacco-control field, by the late 1990s, the strategy that emerged had the appearance of a master plan.

—ɷ— Groundwork Through Research

In 1991, Schroeder hired Nancy Kaufman, a registered nurse who holds a graduate degree in administrative and preventive medicine from the University of Wisconsin Medical School, as a vice president. Even more significant, Kaufman, now vice president for philanthropy at Aurora Health Care in Milwaukee, had been deputy director of public health in Wisconsin and brought to the Foundation's Princeton, New Jersey, headquarters a finely tuned political sense. Although Wisconsin is not generally thought of as a tobacco state, its farmers do produce tobacco for wrappers and chewing tobacco, and Kaufman had considerable experience with tobacco-control issues. Hughes, Kaufman, and their colleagues working on tobacco realized that the first priority was to build a foundation of evidenced-based science.

Before the Foundation began investing in tobacco-related policy research, most researchers in the field were involved in epidemiological questions—patterns of use and cancer rates. The Foundation wanted to focus its research dollars on assessments of public- and private-sector policies that can affect tobacco use—such as regulation, taxes, and reducing young people's access to tobacco—to gauge their feasibility and effectiveness and to educate decision makers about the results. In January 1992, the Foundation's board of trustees approved $5 million over two years to establish the Tobacco Policy Research and Evaluation Program, or TPREP. Two years later, the board authorized an expansion of the policy research component to include alcohol

Table 1.1 Tobacco-Control Grants of Over $1 Million

Title	Institution	Start	End	Amount
Section A: Tobacco National Program Initiatives				
SmokeLess States: National Tobacco Policy Initiative	American Medical Association	05/01/93	12/31/04	$99,000,000
National Center for Tobacco-Free Kids	National Center for Tobacco-Free Kids	02/01/96	01/31/07	$84,000,000
Smoke-Free Families: Innovations to Stop Smoking During and Beyond Pregnancy	University of Alabama at Birmingham School of Medicine	05/01/93	04/30/07	$23,413,278
Substance Abuse Policy Research Program	Center for Creative Leadership	08/01/94	06/30/07	$13,368,895
Partners with Tobacco Use Research Centers: Advancing Transdisciplinary Science and Policy Studies	University of Illinois at Chicago	05/01/99	03/31/07	$12,504,070
Smoking Cessation Leadership Center	University of California, San Francisco	11/01/02	01/31/08	$10,000,000
National Tobacco Control Technical Assistance Consortium	Emory University, Rollins School of Public Health	02/01/01	09/30/04	$7,198,187
Research Network on the Etiology of Tobacco Dependence	University of Kentucky, Center for Prevention Research	02/01/96	09/30/04	$7,886,778
Helping Young Smokers Quit: Identifying Best Practices for Tobacco Cessation	University of Illinois at Chicago	08/01/01	07/31/06	$7,500,000
Addressing Tobacco in Managed Care	University of Wisconsin Medical School	11/01/96	04/30/05	$6,447,141
Tobacco Policy Research and Evaluation Program	Stanford University School of Law	02/01/92	10/31/96	$4,593,490
Bridging the Gap: Research Informing Practice for Healthy Youth Behavior	University of Illinois at Chicago	08/01/97	02/28/06	$4,559,520
Policy Advocacy on Tobacco and Health: An Initiative to Build Capacity in Communities of Color for Tobacco Policy Change	The Praxis Project Inc.	05/01/02	08/31/05	$3,800,000
Innovators Combating Substance Abuse	Johns Hopkins University School of Medicine	05/01/98	11/30/06	$1,750,000
Developing Leadership in Reducing Substance Abuse	Portland State University, Graduate School of Social Work	05/01/98	02/28/07	$1,500,000

Section B: Ad-hoc Grants over $1 Million

Project	Organization			Amount
Why Youth Don't Quit: Finding answers to design effective smoking cessation programs	Health Research, Inc.	03/01/02	02/28/06	$3,499,508
Voices in the Debate: Minority Action for Tobacco Policy Change	Association of Asian Pacific Community Health Organizations	09/01/01	08/31/06	$2,500,000
Voices in the Debate: Minority Action for Tobacco Policy Change	National Latino Council on Alcohol and Tobacco Prevention	07/01/01	06/30/06	$2,500,000
Statewide Youth-led Program to Prevent Tobacco Use by Young People	State of North Carolina Department of Health and Human Services	11/01/99	07/31/04	$1,993,698
Tobacco-Free Nurses: Helping nurses quit	University of California, Los Angeles, School of Nursing	08/01/03	07/31/06	$1,800,000
Do National-Level Tobacco Policies Decrease Smoking: A four-country tobacco policy study	Health Research, Inc.	08/01/02	07/31/04	$1,500,000
Four-Community Project to Reduce Adolescent Tobacco Use	Stop Teenage Addiction to Tobacco	09/01/91	12/31/94	$1,246,889
National Center on Addiction and Substance Abuse	National Center on Addiction and Substance Abuse at Columbia University	05/01/97	04/30/05	$20,998,963
Join Together	Boston University School of Public Health	09/01/91	04/30/05	$33,591,683
National Spit Tobacco Education Program—Major League Baseball Initiative	Oral Health America, America's Fund for Dental Health	05/01/96	07/31/05	$10,437,489
Support and Education to the U.S. Public for the Framework Convention on Tobacco Control	National Center for Tobacco-Free Kids	03/01/00	10/31/04	$3,991,235
Planning, Evaluating, and Improving the D.A.R.E. Program	The University of Akron	11/01/99	12/31/05	$3,037,724
Voices in the Debate: Minority Action for Tobacco Policy Change	National African American Tobacco Prevention Network	06/01/02	03/31/07	$2,426,059
The 11th World Conference on Tobacco OR Health	American Medical Association	05/01/96	12/31/02	$1,994,339
PRISM Awards: Encouraging accurate depictions of substance abuse and addiction in entertainment industry products	Entertainment Industries Council Inc.	12/15/98	06/14/04	$1,959,093
Section C: Ad-hoc Grants Less Than $1 Million—Total				$65,400,015
Total				$446,398,054

and illicit drugs, and with a three-year, $11 million grant, the Substance Abuse Policy Research Program, or SAPRP, was formed.[8]

In addition to spotlighting effective policy alternatives, the programs were charged with "growing the field" of tobacco-policy research—which was relatively small at the time. With its steady stream of funding, TPREP and SAPRP hoped to attract researchers from a wide variety of disciplines, including medicine, public health, law, sociology, political science, and psychology, to conduct tobacco policy research. They succeeded. About 25 percent of the researchers supported by early TPREP grants reported in interviews that they were relatively new to the field of tobacco-policy research.[9]

This marriage of research and policy analysis quickly yielded results. Some of the early findings helped lay the groundwork in two important policy areas: first, an analysis of the effect of the price of cigarettes on consumption, and, second, an analysis of whether tobacco met the legal definition of a drug. With a TPREP grant, Frank Chaloupka at the University of Illinois at Chicago was able to show that higher prices reduced smoking among teenagers and young adults. This line of research helped shape the argument for higher cigarette excise taxes, which became a key tool for tobacco-control advocates.

Another critical finding, which grew out of the work of John Slade of St. Peter's Medical Center (now St. Peter's University Hospital) and the University of Medicine and Dentistry of New Jersey, bolstered efforts to define nicotine as a drug. Slade collected and sifted through court documents, patents, papers written by tobacco-industry scientists, industry newsletters, and other public documents, looking for evidence on whether tobacco fit the legal definition of a drug. His analysis helped staff members at the Food and Drug Administration to better understand that tobacco products are similar to pharmaceuticals.[10] In August 1996, when the FDA published a final ruling proposing that it regulate nicotine as a drug, it cited Slade's extensive commentary in support of its action.

Not only did the Foundation's investment in tobacco-policy research yield important findings but it also came at a critical time for the emerging discipline. "The program put tobacco policy on the map," said Kenneth Warner, a health economist at the University of Michigan School of Public Health. "There was only a handful of researchers, and we were in a sort of hand-to-mouth existence. We found it interesting, but it was not where the money was. Once SAPRP was established, it attracted new, first-rate researchers who had never done tobacco research before."

—w— The Policy and Advocacy Piece

As the sphere of tobacco-policy researchers expanded, the Foundation turned its attention to marshaling the fruits of that research to advocate for policy changes to curb tobacco use. Kaufman asked Michael Beachler, then a senior program officer at the Foundation, to help devise an advocacy structure that would take full advantage of the growing body of policy research. They recommended that the Foundation support coalitions of tobacco-control organizations that would be largely immune from the influence of the tobacco industry. In 1993, The Robert Wood Johnson Foundation authorized a $10 million grant to establish the SmokeLess States program to help the coalitions—often housed in organizations such as the American Cancer Society, the American Heart Association, or the American Lung Association—develop statewide plans and activities to reduce tobacco use, especially among children and teenagers.[11]

Finding the right collaborator was crucial to the success of Smoke-Less States. Schroeder, who rarely involved himself in substance-abuse strategy decisions, suggested the American Medical Association as the Foundation's partner. Since lobbying would be necessary to counter the influence of the tobacco industry and, by federal law, the Foundation was precluded from doing so, the Foundation insisted that its SmokeLess States grantees find matching money from other sources. This turned out to be a great incentive for the SmokeLess States coalitions to raise funds.

In 2000, the focus of the SmokeLess States program was changed, and state coalitions were required to concentrate exclusively on policies that would reduce smoking. At its apex, SmokeLess States had statewide coalitions in forty-two states that focused on policy changes in the areas of increased excise taxes on tobacco, clean indoor air, and reimbursement for costs of cessation and treatment programs. The coalitions also challenged public officials to deter tobacco use through legislative means. In

West Virginia, for example, a SmokeLess States coalition trained teenagers to become antismoking peer advocates and funded tobacco-control chapters throughout the state. Today more than 80 percent of the state's counties have clean indoor air ordinances and teenage tobacco use has declined significantly.[12] In Montana, the coalition's efforts contributed to passage of a groundbreaking clean-air ordinance in Helena in 2002. It also helped organize an effort that resulted in an increase in excise taxes from eighteen cents—one of the nation's lowest rates—to seventy cents. In Massachusetts, the SmokeLess States coalition's work led to the state government's raising the tax on cigarettes to $1.51 a carton, once the highest in the nation.

—∿— The Center for Tobacco-Free Kids: A Counterweight to the Tobacco Industry

Kaufman was a member of the Foundation's delegation to the 1994 World Conference on Tobacco OR Health, in Paris. For her—and, as it turned out, for the Foundation—it was a pivotal moment. Surrounded by a global group of advocates, academics, and government officials, she was stunned by how far behind the United States was in developing coherent tobacco-control policies. Between sessions, a group of tobacco-control advocates, including Matt Myers, a Washington-based attorney and antismoking advocate, began discussing the need for a national center that could operate as a central command post for the fragmented antismoking forces in the United States. At the time, the Coalition on Smoking OR Health, a loose confederation of the American Cancer Society, the American Lung Association, and the American Heart Association, was the movement's only voice, but it was underfunded and mainly just reacted to the tobacco industry's media campaigns.

The antismoking partisans in Paris agreed that a national center needed to be more than just a communications shop. Beyond ministering to the press and providing information, documentation, and sound bites for the tobacco-control point of view, it would push for policy change to denormalize tobacco. Its foe—albeit a kind of David-and-Goliath matchup—was the formidable Tobacco Institute, the multimillion-dollar public-relations behemoth whose thirty-six year run of fending off the mounting scientific evidence of tobacco's adverse impact on the nation's health was the stuff of legend. Back in Princeton, Kaufman and Beachler made their pitch to Schroeder. He approved the concept, and what would arguably become the Foundation's preeminent tobacco-control entity began to take shape.

Within The Robert Wood Johnson Foundation, this overt and highly visible confrontation with the tobacco industry was viewed as a controversial step. To confirm that the idea of a national antismoking center was in keeping with the Foundation's focus on smoking among young people, the new national tobacco-control clearinghouse was named the National Center for Tobacco-Free Kids. Funding partners were enlisted to join the fight. In the fall of 1995, the American Cancer Society and the American Heart Association made five-year financial commitments to the project. The following January, The Robert Wood Johnson Foundation authorized a grant of $20 million. (In 1999, a renewal grant of $50 million was approved for the period April 1999 to March 2004. Its third, and last, grant is for $14 million, which expires in 2007.)

The Center opened for business shortly after Labor Day 1995. In August, the White House and the FDA had announced the federal government's intention to assert jurisdiction over tobacco, ushering in an era of unprecedented government attention to tobacco-control efforts. William D. Novelli, a founder of the social marketing and public relations firm of Porter Novelli, was intercepted as he was about to take a sabbatical at the Annenberg School for Communication at the University of Pennsylvania after stepping down from the position of executive vice president at CARE. He became the Center's first president. Matt Myers, one of the strategists at the Paris conference, officially joined the Center as vice president at its official opening in June 1996. (He is now the organization's president.)

The Center has four goals: to develop a national strategy for reducing youth tobacco use, to serve as a media and information center to parry the tobacco industry's promotional thrusts, to provide technical assistance to state and community antismoking education efforts, and to broaden the base of national organization support to reduce youth tobacco use.

In 1999, the Center launched the Campaign for Tobacco-Free Kids and developed a National Action Network, including more than 300,000 grassroots members ready to speak out on issues regarding youth tobacco use. It has allied with more than 142 health, civic, educational, youth, and religious groups dedicated to reducing tobacco use among children. The Center sponsors two nationally recognized events—Kick Butts Day and the Youth Advocates of the Year Awards. Kick Butts Day, held every April, features more than 1,500 events in all fifty states and abroad, involving elementary, middle school, and high school students speaking out against the marketing of tobacco to kids and taking action in their communities.

A Web site, www.tobaccofreekids.org, informs the public, policymakers, and the media about tobacco control and other ways for these groups to become involved in the effort. The Web site carries the full texts of the Center's fact sheets, press releases, advertisements, and special reports. A recent special report, for example, lists campaign contributions made by tobacco companies to every senator and representative. The Center seeks to broaden public and institutional support for state-level policy change, such as increasing state excise taxes on tobacco products, expanding protections against secondary smoke, and assuring that states will use their money from the $209 billion settlement with the tobacco industry for comprehensive prevention programs. The Center also is working to broaden public support for the regulation of tobacco by the FDA.

Shortly after opening, the Center was presented with a difficult—and its most wrenching—decision. A number of states had filed suits seeking to recoup the cost of treatment for cancer victims that had been paid for by state Medicaid funds, and in early 1996 Novelli and Myers were asked to act as a liaison with the public health community.[13] In March 1997, the tobacco industry was hinting at a deal, and the White House wanted Myers and the Center to be present during the negotiations. Once the talks were reported by the *Wall Street Journal* in April, the Center came under heavy fire from militant antismoking activists for sitting down with the tobacco industry—an act that many construed as a betrayal.

The talks led to a historic agreement in June 1997, obligating the industry to make annual payments to the states estimated to total nearly $370 billion in the first twenty-five years and to continue indefinitely. It also gave the FDA authority to regulate tobacco, curtailed tobacco marketing, limited ads in magazines with large youth readership, and set aside funds to be used for tobacco cessation and treatment efforts. With money raised privately by the Center, Myers began working with Senator John McCain's office to get enabling legislation passed. It was introduced in March 1998 and died by filibuster in June of that year. In November, a new but weaker agreement was announced—the Master Settlement Agreement—that was a disappointment to the antismoking camp. Key aspects of the earlier agreement, such as FDA authority over tobacco, standards for secondhand smoke, tougher warnings on tobacco products, and penalties for tobacco companies if youth smoking rates did not decline, had been lost.[14]

After the Master Settlement Agreement, the National Center for Tobacco-Free Kids increased its focus on the states, where the Foundation's SmokeLess States program and other state and local advocate groups were ready to wage battles over funding for prevention and cessation programs, protection from secondhand smoke, and increasing excise taxes on tobacco. "From the beginning, the Center saw its role as encouraging federal and state activities in tobacco control and using our communication skills to broaden the movement," Myers said. "The Center's first two years were focused on the settlement and legislation. But over the last four to five years, our attention has been focused on becoming a resource for state and local efforts and to make sure they are as integrated as possible. We work to see that the many Robert Wood Johnson Foundation projects in different areas are integrated into the related efforts of others so that the projects are seen not as a thousand points of light but as an integrated whole greater than the sum of its parts."

—⁓— Treatment and Cessation Programs

As the senior scientist at The Robert Wood Johnson Foundation, C. Tracy Orleans has played a leadership role in developing the grantmaking strategy in the area of tobacco-dependence treatment. Like many others at the Foundation, she had personal reasons for being interested in tobacco. "I had a terrible time quitting," Orleans recalled. "That experience really focused me on treatment and cessation programs."

Tobacco-policy research in the early 1990s had shown the benefits of certain cessation approaches, namely counseling and pharmaceuticals, but not many physicians or health care organizations were actively employing these tools. In 1996, the federal Agency for Health Care Policy and Research (now the Agency for Healthcare Research and Quality) identified effective treatments that could reduce tobacco-related disease and death dramatically—such as counseling by a physician and the use of pharmacological agents—and issued guidelines for their use. As a logical next step, the Foundation sought to capitalize on the guidelines by seeking to make them a regular part of medical practice, particularly within managed-care systems.

While managed-care organizations should benefit from encouraging healthy lifestyles and emphasizing preventive medicine, their constantly changing membership—which meant that they might not reap the economic benefit of their investments in prevention—slowed the adoption of tobacco-cessation treatments. The Foundation hoped that its investments in treatment and cessation would help translate science into medical practice—always a slow and difficult process. The staff also had to weigh the grantmaking trade-offs between prevention and treatment.

Orleans felt that the tobacco-control strategy had to embrace both spheres: "We needed a multipronged approach—one that combines 'upstream' efforts to promote environmental change through education and policy change, with more 'downstream' efforts to identify and disseminate effective prevention and treatment programs."[15] She observed the great gap between "what we know and what we do."[16] Only 50 to 60 percent of smokers report getting any advice on quitting from their physicians. Fewer than 25 percent report any further counseling or drug-based therapy. Low-income and minority smokers are the least likely to get this help.

Why the gap has not narrowed is due to a number of factors: lack of training in medical school, doctors underestimating the difficulty in overcoming tobacco addiction, health care systems not supporting cessation efforts, insurance and reimbursement policies not covering tobacco-dependence treatment, weak demand for such services by smokers, and the lack of a strong "business case" for treatment.[17]

With these realities in mind, the Foundation decided on two goals for its cessation efforts: identifying and promoting effective tobacco-cessation treatments and translating them into clinical practice. To reach those goals, the staff devised a three-part strategy: bolstering the scientific basis for tobacco-dependent treatment, strengthening the capacity of health care systems to deliver effective intervention, and building a market and demand for effective treatments among health care providers, purchasers, policymakers, and consumers.

To give managed care organizations an incentive to offer tobacco-cessation counseling and treatment, the Foundation targeted the report cards issued by the National Committee on Quality Assurance, a Washington, D.C.–based organization that provides information on quality and cost of medical care to managed care plans. These report cards, officially known as Health Plan Employer Data and Information Set, or HEDIS, are used by health care buyers, such as corporations, when selecting health plans for their employees. In 1996, a tobacco-reporting component—based on whether HMO-enrolled smokers had been advised to quit in the past year—was included in HEDIS. It marked the first time that a behavioral risk factor was made part of the annual evaluations.

One of the Foundation's major cessation programs, Addressing Tobacco in Managed Care, offers a good illustration of the complexities of persuading clinicians to adopt cessation practices. The program, launched in 1997, asked managed care organizations and their academic partners to submit research ideas on how the federal smoking-cessation guidelines could be woven into health care settings. The premise was that managed care organizations are ideally situated to incorporate tobacco interventions in everyday clinical practice because they have access to enrolled populations and can provide incentives, tools, and structural support to their provider networks.

According to a 2001 evaluation of Addressing Tobacco in Managed Care done by the Schneider Institute for Health Policy at Brandeis University, the program has had mixed results.[18] Evaluators found that the program had "created an air of awareness" in the minds of managed care organizations, researchers, and providers about tobacco dependence, had built up the field's knowledge about the issue, and had created collaborations among academics, new researchers, and managed care organizations. Yet the evaluation team also reported some characteristics inherent in the health care system that worked against the effort. While the Addressing Tobacco in Managed Care program framed tobacco dependence as a chronic recurring disease, the managed care organizations tended to regard it as a health promotion issue. This view led them away from locating tobacco-dependence efforts in clinical settings, where they had the most potential rewards, and instead putting them in the hands of the marketing and/or quality improvement departments.

—w— A Look Back on the Tobacco Strategy

For Americans of a certain age, the widespread condemnation of the tobacco industry, the near universal expectation of clean indoor air, the *de rigeur* disapproval of youth smoking, the transformation of smoking from a cool, Hollywood-fueled affectation to a reckless, inexplicable, and disheartening personal choice is nothing short of a sea change in social values and behavior. Not many decades ago, small, complimentary packs of cigarettes would appear alongside the entree on many commercial airline flights. Nowadays, huge numbers of people have quit, or are trying to, and the tobacco companies themselves are spending millions on ads asking, perhaps disingenuously, kids not to smoke.

In the 1990s, when the Foundation entered the fray, many factors had intertwined to help bring about this shift: the Surgeon General's report; the work of advocacy groups; the growing media attention to the hazards of smoking; lawsuits filed against the tobacco companies by lung cancer victims; and legislation on the federal, state, and local levels to protect innocent people from secondhand smoke. What, then, was the role of The Robert Wood Johnson Foundation in this remarkable and remarkably complex company of actors in the tobacco-control crusade?

From the vantage point of 2004, Schroeder, who now heads the Smoking Cessation Leadership Center at the University of California, San Francisco, offered this opinion on the Foundation's tobacco-control work:

"In general, I didn't know what to expect, but as a portfolio we probably outperformed where we thought we could go."

But outperformed against what measure? It is impossible to quantify, beyond some positive trends, how the Foundation's investments paid off. But its entrance and, perhaps more important, its steady presence in the field of tobacco control has unquestionably had a significant impact on a difficult and insidious health issue.

Michael Pertschuk, the former chairman of the Federal Trade Commission and cofounder and codirector of the Advocacy Institute in Washington, D.C., has had a long career in public health and an abiding interest in tobacco control. (He also has written a book, *Smoke in Their Eyes: Lessons in Movement Leadership from the Tobacco Wars*, funded by The Robert Wood Johnson Foundation.) To Pertschuk, the Foundation helped transform the field by moving shrewdly and decisively and with unprecedented resources. "It was probably the biggest player, but size was not as important as its strategic focus," Pertschuk said. "As The Robert Wood Johnson Foundation began to get involved in tobacco control, it did so with an understanding that it would not be just more social marketing, but attempts at systemic change. It had to take on the fundamental political dimension of the problem. It was a unique strategic intervention in the public health field that will serve as a model for years to come." In terms of its influence, Pertschuk says, "The Foundation can certainly claim credit for decreases in youth smoking and arresting the late '90s upward trend among young smokers, and they were dominant in their role as a provider of strategic resources to the field, particularly with communications guidance, media support and polling. On the state level, they brought cohesion to the advocacy network—in a field that previously had no full-time staff working solely on tobacco."

Just as important—to researchers, at least—is how the Foundation almost single-handedly brought the tobacco research community to scale. David Altman, the program director of both the Tobacco Policy Research and Evaluation Program and Substance Abuse Policy Research Program, remembered how the field used to be. "In the mid- to late-1980s people were beginning to talk about doing research in tobacco," he said. "But at the time there were maybe fifteen people in the whole country who were interested in that kind of work. Once The Robert Wood Johnson Foundation began to offer research grants, it almost instantly legitimized the field."

Similarly, Susan Curry, codirector of the Addressing Tobacco in Managed Care program, believes that the Foundation's investments to promote the most promising tobacco cessation and treatment practices in managed care organizations has had an even greater and more long-lasting effect. "It's my firm belief that because of the progress on tobacco in managed care, the health care community is now addressing the bigger concept of treating health-risk behaviors, be it tobacco use, poor nutrition, or physical inactivity," she said.

It is not surprising to hear such glowing report cards from those populating the Foundation's far-flung tobacco-control activities. Yet critics of the National Center for Tobacco-Free Kids' involvement in the settlement talks remain unforgiving, and others in the field find much to complain about in the Foundation's approach and many of its key assumptions. One of the Foundation's most vociferous critics is Stanton Glantz, professor of medicine and the director of the Center for Tobacco Control Research and Education at the University of California, San Francisco (and a recipient of a Robert Wood Johnson Innovators in Substance Abuse Award in 2002). A straight-talking, pragmatic veteran of the tobacco wars, Glantz recalls, somewhat wistfully, that at one time he lobbied the Foundation to enter the field. "It was a case of 'beware of what you wish for,'" he says. "The need for a major foundation to get involved was long overdue, and there's no question that the Foundation had a very strong agenda-setting role. It's just that a number of things they did were wrong."

The Foundation's focus on youth smoking, Glantz believes, was a bad decision that diverted time and money away from other more effective targets, namely, in Glantz's view, clean indoor air and tobacco tax policy. "The companies themselves were focused on kids smoking, and it was politically safer for the Foundation to concentrate on children," he said. "But they got the whole movement derailed on youth access and preventing the first cigarette. They fell into that trap and did not pay enough attention to where the real power was: bottom-up, grassroots advocacy on clean indoor air. Their whole model and mentality was East Coast, Washingtoncentric, and top-down. But the National Center for Tobacco-Free Kids is not where the action is; it's always at the local and state level. The further you go up the political tree, the more money talks, the more lobbyists talk, the more lawyers talk. And the tobacco companies have lots of money, lobbyists, and lawyers."

Glantz goes on to fault the Foundation's Washington D.C.–based tobacco-control generals for being heavy-handed in issuing directives. "The fight for nonsmokers' rights should be driven by what people want, not what a bunch of graybeards want," he said. "Their notion of a grassroots campaign was an e-mail action campaign, *telling* people what to do."

As for the National Center for Tobacco-Free Kids' involvement in the tobacco settlement, Glantz is squarely in the camp seeing it as a huge blunder. "There was a big split between those in D.C. who thought it necessary to give the tobacco industry significant concessions versus the people in the field who had sent tobacco packing on indoor air fights and knew what it was like to have a clean victory," he said. "The brokering of the settlement was in direct opposition to everybody else and did great damage to the whole movement. It destroyed a lot of relationships, and it was wrong strategically and at a policy level."

Taking the long view, even as harsh a critic as Glantz sees the Foundation's tobacco strategy as having ripened with age as it moved toward the less centralized state-based advocacy efforts that he favors. "They went through a ten-year learning curve, but in the last three years or so they were just over the hump and getting some traction. In another ten years, if they did it right, like they were beginning to do it, they could have wiped tobacco out." With characteristic candor, he concludes: "They put tobacco control on the public agenda but wasted a huge amount of energy and money doing so. After ten years, they finally got it right and created a potent infrastructure, and then they walked away."

Bearing such criticisms in mind, after more than a dozen years of grantmaking and hundreds of millions of dollars in investments how should the Foundation's engagement in the tobacco wars be judged? A reasoned interpretation of all the evidence leads to a positive conclusion. The Robert Wood Johnson Foundation entered the tobacco-control arena with superb timing and had an enormous catalyzing effect, reenergizing existing tobacco-control forces and playing a crucial role in the development of new approaches. With a sustained flow of financial resources to all corners of the field and an overall strategy that coalesced into a proven and effective integrated battle plan, the Foundation can take significant credit for one of the major public health triumphs in recent years. As Schroeder and others concede, the Foundation's now widely admired tobacco-control strategy came together in bits and pieces. But seen in retrospect, it could rightfully be held up as a model—blending policy research, state-based advocacy and coalition building, and a national communications and strategic command center—for others seeking social change against formidable odds.

—∿— Winding Down

Risa Lavizzo-Mourey took over as president of The Robert Wood Johnson Foundation in 2003. As was true of Schroeder twelve years earlier, Lavizzo-Mourey was eager to put her own stamp on the Foundation. A geriatrician with clinical experience in chronic illness, she had been a Robert Wood Johnson Clinical Scholar. As she and the board reviewed the Foundation's direction, it became clear that Lavizzo-Mourey had plans to reduce investments in some areas—notably, end-of-life care and tobacco—and redeploy them.

In an interview posted on the Foundation's Web site, Lavizzo-Mourey elaborated on her rationale. Expressing pride in what the staff and the grantees have accomplished in reducing the use of tobacco, Lavizzo-Mourey explained, "The reason we are trying to balance our prevention efforts is that there are now new threats on the horizon. We have seen some decrease in the prevalence of smoking, so we can and should shift some of our attention to these new threats. We try to look at areas where there is a significant need." She elaborated, "When you look at the causes of preventable mortality in this country, smoking and tobacco use rival lack of physical activity and obesity for the number one and number two slots. Many of the chronic diseases that plague us, like cardiovascular disease, hypertension, diabetes, stroke, and many cancers, are related to those two unhealthy behaviors. If you look at the epidemiology, you see that obesity, particularly obesity in children, is becoming more common, and there's a decline in physical activity associated with that rise in obesity. Consistent with our mission [of improving health and health care], we need to focus our prevention resources on the areas that are the biggest threats. In addition to the work that we've invested in reducing the harm caused by tobacco over the years, we think it's important to add obesity, particularly among children, to that prevention portfolio."

Lavizzo-Mourey took pains in the interview to insist that the Foundation would not become complacent about the risks of tobacco and would remain vigilant in not only maintaining hard-won gains but also making further progress in smoking cessation and in helping people resist starting. "We will not abandon tobacco- and substance abuse-related prevention," she said, "but we would be remiss if we didn't pay attention to obesity, another grave and growing threat."

The Foundation's plan going forward, Lavizzo-Mourey said, is to sustain the tobacco-control policy infrastructure and its research base through a cluster of programs, projects, and communications activities. She projected a $72 million grantmaking budget for tobacco control over the next two years and $30 million more through 2008. She also said that if trends started "going in the wrong direction," the Foundation would reconsider its funding decisions.

The reduced emphasis on tobacco control has, predictably, raised concerns. "The phaseout of tobacco was a very difficult decision," said the Foundation's Robert Hughes, "but we are doing it in a responsible way. We are doing no harm because we are retaining the structures, and retaining a commitment to the field. But, yes, there is a very real risk of losing some gains. We would have a much less healthy population were it not for the work the Foundation has done. The question is, will the phaseout come at a price to the public's health and can the investments in childhood obesity compensate?"

Other experts in tobacco control express similar fears. "I have to respect each new president's vision, and I applaud Risa on her attention to obesity in children," said Kenneth Warner, the University of Michigan health economist. "But I am terribly disappointed by the lack of resources [for tobacco research]. If you look back on the last decade, the first part was the most exciting, but the most recent year was the most depressing, because all the resources that took so long to build up are being dissipated."

The phaseout coincides with tough budget times for the states, and the Advocacy Institute's Mike Pertschuk sees that as a double whammy affecting the state-based antismoking coalitions. "If you didn't have the simultaneous plunge in funding in the states, it wouldn't be so threatening, because the leadership is mature and well-established," he said. "But you can't say that now. In terms of its timing, in the setting of state economic crises, the phaseout is a serious blow." Pertschuk is more sanguine about other aspects of the tobacco control. "There seems to be strong, independent momentum for smoke-free environments, and the same goes for tax increases. Cessation activities will suffer somewhat, and on the national level there is still a major need for the Center for Tobacco-Free Kids."

Mindful of the tricky course she must navigate going forward, Lavizzo-Mourey is pragmatic. In the Internet interview, she said, "We know that we cannot do everything. To take on something like tobacco or obesity requires not only a major financial commitment, but also intellectual commitment, passion for the work on our part, and collaboration to leverage other resources from people around the country. There are only so many big issues you can take on at a time, and no foundation can take any of them on unilaterally. . . . What are the most pressing for us to engage in right now? That's going to change over time. And frankly, the amount of the resources that we put into any one will also change over time as the environment—the external forces with which we contend—change. The only way to keep this in balance is to keep asking ourselves what are the most pressing issues and how can we use our resources most effectively to make a difference?"

Notes

1. Hughes, R. "Adopting the Substance Abuse Goal." *To Improve Health and Health Care 1998–1999: The Robert Wood Johnson Foundation Anthology.* San Francisco: Jossey-Bass, 1999.

2. Schapiro, R. "A Conversation with Steven Schroeder." *To Improve Health and Health Care, Vol. VI: The Robert Wood Johnson Foundation Anthology.* San Francisco: Jossey-Bass, 2003.

3. Hughes, R. "Adopting the Substance Abuse Goal." *To Improve Health and Health Care 1998–1999: The Robert Wood Johnson Foundation Anthology.* San Francisco: Jossey-Bass, 1999.

4. http://www.cdc.gov/tobacco/overview/oshsummary2004.htm

5. *Substance Abuse, The Nation's Number One Health Problem: Key Indicators for Policy.* Prepared by the Schneider Institute for Health Policy, Brandeis University, for The Robert Wood Johnson Foundation, February 2001.

6. The Center for Tobacco Free Kids (http://tobaccofreekids.org/research/factsheets/pdf/0002.pdf).

7. Koppett, L. "The National Spit Tobacco Education Program." *To Improve Health and Health Care 1998–1999: The Robert Wood Johnson Foundation Anthology.* San Francisco: Jossey-Bass, 1999.

8. Gutman, M. A., Altman, D. G., and Rabin, R. L. "Tobacco Policy Research." *To Improve Health and Health Care 1998–1999: The Robert Wood Johnson Foundation Anthology.* San Francisco: Jossey-Bass, 1999.

9. The Lewin Group. *Assessment of the Substance Abuse Policy Research Program and Tobacco Policy Research and Evaluation Program.* Fairfax, Va.: The Lewin Group, 1997.

10. Gutman, M. A., Altman, D. G., and Rabin, R. L. "Tobacco Policy Research." *To Improve Health and Health Care 1998–1999: The Robert Wood Johnson Foundation Anthology.* San Francisco: Jossey-Bass, 1999.

11. See Chapter Two in this volume.

12. http://ama-assn.org/ama/pub/print/article/3216–7745.html

13. See Diehl, D. "The Center for Tobacco-Free Kids and the Tobacco-Settlement Negotiations." *To Improve Health and Health Care, Vol. VI: The Robert Wood Johnson Foundation Anthology.* San Francisco: Jossey-Bass, 2003.

14. Schroeder, S. A. "Tobacco Control in the Wake of the 1998 Master Settlement Agreement." *New England Journal of Medicine,* 2004, *350,* 293–301.

15. Orleans, C. T. "Challenges and Opportunities for Tobacco Control: The Robert Wood Johnson Foundation Agenda." *Tobacco Control,* 1998, *7*(Supp.), S8–S11.

16. Orleans, C. T., and Alper, J. "Helping Addicted Smokers Quit." *To Improve Health and Health Care, Vol. VI: The Robert Wood Johnson Foundation Anthology.* San Francisco: Jossey-Bass, 2003.

17. Ibid.

18. *Addressing Tobacco in Managed Care, An Evaluative Assessment.* Schneider Institute for Health Policy, Brandeis University, January 2001.

2

The SmokeLess States Program

Karen K. Gerlach and Michelle A. Larkin

Editors' Introduction

Through the SmokeLess States Program, The Robert Wood Johnson Foundation has supported the work of state tobacco-control coalitions across the nation. The program ranks among the largest investments ever made by the Foundation, with $99 million authorized since 1992—more than a fifth of the Foundation's $420 million portfolio of grants designed to reduce tobacco use in the United States.

In this chapter, Karen Gerlach and Michelle Larkin, the two program officers currently responsible for overseeing the SmokeLess States Program, chronicle its development, implementation, and impact. Two features about the program stand out. First, the Foundation encouraged its grantees (state tobacco-control coalitions) to be activists—to try to bring about social change rather than doing research to find out how social change can be brought about. Second, and following from the first, the Foundation unabashedly emphasized advocacy to bring about policy change. The authors trace the program's evolution from one with both educational and advocacy elements to one focused exclusively on advocacy.

This meant that the Foundation had to be especially careful that its funds not be used for lobbying. It provided training to grantees and monitored the program vigilantly to be sure that federal laws prohibiting the use of foundation funds for lobbying were scrupulously followed.

The SmokeLess States program relied on an approach to social change traditionally taken by The Robert Wood Johnson Foundation—the support of coalitions.[1] Thus, in addition to its insights on the role of advocacy, this chapter offers a window into the role of coalitions in bringing about social change.

The chapter complements the one by James Bornemeier in this year's *Robert Wood Johnson Foundation Anthology* that reviews the Foundation's investments to reduce the harm caused by tobacco.[2]

1. See, for example, Wielawski, I. "The Fighting Back Program." *To Improve Health and Health Care, Vol. VII: The Robert Wood Johnson Foundation Anthology.* San Francisco: Jossey-Bass, 2004; and Jellinek, P., and Schapiro, R. "Join Together and CADCA: Backing Up the Front Line." *To Improve Health and Health Care, Vol. VII: The Robert Wood Johnson Foundation Anthology.* San Francisco: Jossey-Bass, 2004.
2. Chapter One in this volume.

P rior to the early 1990s, The Robert Wood Johnson Foundation had not addressed the threat that tobacco use posed to life and health in the United States. Most of the Foundation's grantmaking had focused on improving the delivery of health care services. Those limited investments that had been made to improve health were largely directed toward preventing the use of illicit drugs.[1]

When Steven Schroeder became the third president of The Robert Wood Johnson Foundation in 1990, he arrived with the understanding that the Foundation could not help to improve the health of all Americans unless it addressed the harm caused by tobacco. Even before taking office, Schroeder had made clear to the Foundation's board of trustees his desire to make tobacco a significant new area of the Foundation's grantmaking.[2] At the time, tobacco use caused 400,000 deaths a year.

—ᴿ— The SmokeLess States Program Takes Shape

In 1992, the trustees authorized the development of programs that would curb the use of tobacco, especially among young people for whom smoking was illegal.[3] Schroeder designated Nancy Kaufman, a public health professional from Wisconsin, who had recently joined the Foundation as a vice president, to design the Foundation's tobacco-control programs, and Kaufman in turn asked Michael Beachler, who was a program officer with experience in health policy, to assist her. They worked under the umbrella of a Foundation group headed by Robert Hughes that was developing programs to curb substance abuse, including tobacco.

As one of its initial investments, the Foundation funded the Tobacco Policy Research and Evaluation Program, which supported research to examine policies that might have an impact on tobacco use—such as research demonstrating the link between cigarette excise taxes and reduced smoking rates.[4] Understanding the policies that might affect tobacco use was an essential first step. Translating that evidence into practice was an important second step. Kaufman asked Beachler to determine how best to do this, and suggested that he familiarize himself with work going on in

California—at that time the only state that had allocated substantial resources to tobacco control. Following the passage of its Proposition 99 in 1988, which imposed a tax on tobacco products and dedicated the revenue to addressing tobacco use, California designed and adopted a comprehensive program to reduce smoking throughout the state. The program included countermarketing, cessation services, research, and prevention efforts. After spending time in California and observing how the state was spending its tobacco tax funds, Beachler concluded that the California experiment was tailor-made for a Robert Wood Johnson Foundation demonstration program in which a variety of approaches could be tried in different states.

To be sure that a new demonstration program would not duplicate other programs, especially the National Cancer Institute's American Stop Smoking Intervention Study, or ASSIST, Beachler attended a meeting of ASSIST grantees. He found that ASSIST, which supported tobacco-control partnerships in seventeen states, appeared to be reducing tobacco use, and also that the states had only limited resources to pay for efforts to reduce tobacco use. Beachler also met with staff members from the Office on Smoking and Health at the Centers for Disease Control and Prevention, or CDC, to learn about its new investments in tobacco-control efforts in states that were not part of ASSIST. From these meetings, he learned that grantees at state health departments often found it difficult to get the attention of their governor, whose support was crucial to their success.

After reviewing their research and interviews, Foundation staff members concluded that a private-sector voice was needed to complement government-funded programs. They felt that The Robert Wood Johnson Foundation could most effectively translate policy research into policy change by awarding grants to coalitions of nongovernmental organizations that would educate the public and policymakers about the tobacco problem and potential ways to address it. Thus the concept of the Smoke-Less States program was born.

One of the first issues to be faced by The Robert Wood Johnson Foundation staff was the extent to which the Foundation should be involved in advocacy—that is, advocating for tobacco-control policies.

While the Foundation had supported research on policy for many years, it had not worked to bring about changes in policy. Such work would involve taking a step that worried some members of the staff and the board, so the program's emphasis on policy advocacy was not given prominence, even though it was an important component from the beginning.

A second, related issue was that of lobbying. In state capitals across the country, the tobacco industry lobbied, and it lobbied hard. Lobbying by tobacco-control advocates would have to be done to counteract the actions of the tobacco industry. But federal law prohibits private foundations from lobbying, and grantees cannot legally use Foundation funds for that purpose. Legally, the Foundation's grantees were allowed to use their own resources and matching funds raised privately to lobby. Federal regulations permit foundations to support projects that include lobbying, so long as they support only the nonlobbying portion of the project. Thus, the Foundation's conditions of grant expressly prohibited Foundation funds from being used for lobbying.

A third issue was the selection of a National Program Office, or NPO. As the organization that would directly oversee the administration of the grants and provide technical assistance to the grantees, the NPO would play a key role in the program. The NPO had to be a large organization that was on the side of tobacco control, that commanded the respect of the board and the staff alike, that possessed the administrative ability to manage a large program and the wherewithal to provide technical support to sites around the country, and that had the clout to go toe-to-toe with the tobacco industry, if necessary. The staff determined that the American Medical Association, or AMA, had many of these attributes and that it would be the most appropriate place to house the new SmokeLess States program. The AMA was offered the chance to become the NPO, and it accepted the offer.

In April 1993, the Foundation's staff presented the new program, called SmokeLess States: Statewide Tobacco Prevention and Control, to the board of trustees. The board authorized the program for $10 million over four years. Thomas Houston, a physician who had worked for Doctors Ought to Care, an advocacy organization that engaged physicians in the fight against tobacco, and then had become the director of the AMA's

Department of Preventive Medicine and Environmental Health, became the national program director. As his deputy director he recruited Kathleen Harty, who had spent many years with the Department of Health in Minnesota working on tobacco control. Together, Houston and Harty worked with Foundation staff members to give final shape to the program and to guide its first group of grantee states.

—ᴠᴠ— The SmokeLess States Program and Its Early Challenges

The Foundation established three overall objectives for the SmokeLess States program: (1) reducing the number of children and young people who start using tobacco; (2) reducing the number of people who continue using tobacco; and (3) increasing the public's awareness that reducing tobacco use is an important component of any major effort at health care reform. To accomplish these goals, it sought applications from statewide coalitions made up of organizations such as the health voluntaries (the American Cancer Society, the American Heart Association, and the American Lung Association), state medical societies, hospital associations, and others. The coalitions were to conduct public education campaigns, strengthen prevention and treatment capacity, and advocate for tobacco-control policies. To encourage collaboration among the various organizations working on tobacco control within a state, the Foundation allowed only one coalition per state to apply.

Recognizing that state coalitions were in various stages of readiness to take on this work, the Foundation offered two types of grants under the program: a two-year capacity-building grant and a four-year implementation grant. The Foundation staff expected to award ten capacity-building grants averaging $200,000 and eight implementation grants, ranging from $500,000 to $1.2 million each.

To help the Foundation and the NPO staff assess and select grantees, a National Advisory Committee was created. Joseph Califano, the former secretary of the Department of Health, Education and Welfare, served as its first chairman. With the guidance of the National Advisory Committee and the NPO, the Foundation selected nineteen state coalitions for funding: Alaska, Arizona, Colorado, Florida, Illinois, Kansas, New Jersey, Vermont, and West Virginia, each of which was awarded an implementation grant, and Alabama, Georgia, Kentucky, Maryland, Minnesota, Nebraska, Nevada, Oregon, Virginia, and Washington, which received capacity-building grants. Most of the coalitions were housed in one of the three major health voluntaries; two were housed in their state's medical society.

These coalitions, which began their SmokeLess States grants in 1994, addressed tobacco use in different ways. Some focused on educating the public, others on involving young people, still others on public policy; many coalitions worked on a combination of approaches simultaneously. Alaska's coalition, for example, capitalized on the Iditarod dogsled race, working in partnership with event organizers and sponsoring a dogsled musher to educate Alaskans about the harms of tobacco use. New Jersey's coalition concentrated on increasing public support for raising tobacco excise taxes. It used its grant resources to educate the public about tobacco-related harm and the positive impact that higher tobacco taxes have on deterring youth use.

As the coalitions matured, it became clear that they needed assistance understanding the difference between advocacy and public education, which they were legally permitted to do with Foundation funds, and lobbying, which they were not. To make sure that grantees did not violate the prohibition on lobbying with Foundation funds, the Foundation and the NPO provided training and guidance on the difference. In general, direct lobbying involves communications to a legislator reflecting a view on specific legislation while grassroots lobbying involves a communication with the members of the general public that encourages them to take action on specific legislation. Neither type of lobbying can be done using Foundation funds. Advocacy, that is, educating policymakers and the community generally about issues and the measures that can be taken to address them, is not lobbying.

Since the difference is not always crystal clear, the charge of lobbying can be used as a threat by those who oppose what a foundation and its grantees are doing. A case in point occurred in Colorado. The grantee in that state, the Coalition for Tobacco-Free Colorado, was interested in conducting a media campaign to educate the public about the benefits of increasing the price of tobacco as a way to reduce smoking. (A tobacco tax increase was to appear on the November 1994 ballot.) Shortly after an invitation to bid on the contract for the media campaign was sent to various firms, The Robert Wood Johnson Foundation received a letter from Covington & Burling, a well-known Washington, D.C., law firm that represented tobacco companies. This letter, addressed to the Foundation's proposal manager, Ed Robbins, suggested that the Foundation's support for the Colorado coalition crossed the line into activities that were prohibited under the Internal Revenue Code. The letter stated in part:

> Given the sponsors, the context and the timing of the proposed media campaign, there is at the very least a substantial risk that the campaign will fail to qualify as an "educational" activity, or as "nonpartisan analysis, study, or research," within the meaning of the relevant statutes and Treasury regulations. This, obviously, could have adverse tax consequences for the foundation. More to the point, our clients and we would strenuously object to any use of private foundation funds to support what can fairly be viewed here as a lobbying effort, either expressed or implied. This would adversely affect the interests of our clients, and it would also be contrary to the public policies reflected in the Internal Revenue Code restrictions on the use of tax-deductible funds for legislative activity.

After consulting with Sidney Wentz, the chairman of the board of trustees who was himself an attorney, and J. Warren Wood, the Foundation's general counsel, Robbins responded with a brief assurance that the Foundation's funds were being used in accordance with the law. In December 1994, another letter, addressed this time to Wentz, was sent to the Foundation from a congressman representing a tobacco-producing state. The congressman appended to his letter copies of his correspondence with the Internal Revenue Service questioning the Foundation's tax-exempt status and requesting that the IRS investigate the Foundation's use of resources, particularly its tobacco-control investments. Wentz answered the letter, explaining that the Foundation prohibited the use of its funds for lobbying. No Internal Revenue Service action was forthcoming.

—w— The Evolution of the SmokeLess States Program

During the first few years of the SmokeLess States program, the nineteen state coalitions were, by and large, able to develop and maintain coalitions dedicated to reducing smoking and, in the process, to professionalize the tobacco-prevention movement. In the first year of the program (1994–1995), four states—all of which had coalitions funded under the SmokeLess States program—raised their excise taxes on cigarettes. Although each of these coalitions was engaged in an educational campaign about the impact of tobacco taxes on smoking rates, it is unclear, given the short time that they had been Foundation grantees, what role their Foundation support played in the policy gains.

These changes, plus the reductions in youth smoking that were being reported out of California, demonstrated to other states in the program that policy change was possible and that it could be advanced by using a combination of Foundation funds and unrestricted resources. The approach of disseminating scientifically rigorous research on policy (some of which was supported by the Tobacco Policy Research and Evaluation Program) to a general audience demonstrated that policy change was possible and that it could be effective in reducing tobacco use.

In 1996, the staff reviewed the SmokeLess States program and determined that it was continuing to fulfill an important need in the field by focusing attention on changing policies to reduce tobacco use. Before taking the program forward for a renewal, the staff assessed tobacco-control activities occurring throughout the country. For the tobacco-control field, it was an exciting time. On the federal level, the Food and Drug Administration, or FDA, announced that it would regulate advertising and marketing of tobacco products to young people. It also asserted that it had the authority to regulate nicotine as a drug and cigarettes as the delivery device. The ASSIST program still had two years of funding remaining, though it appeared unlikely that it would be renewed. Finally, the CDC was increasing its support for state health departments to work on tobacco prevention and treatment. The activities of the SmokeLess States coalitions complemented these efforts and, in many instances, enabled the state health departments to go beyond the traditional public health education approach and to reach a broader segment of the state's population.

—ᴡᴡ— Program Renewals: Focusing on Tobacco Policy

Increasing federal interest and investment in tobacco-control efforts, rising youth smoking rates, and the SmokeLess States grantees' initial ability to develop functioning coalitions, creative educational campaigns, and increasingly sophisticated policy advocacy prompted the Foundation staff to request a $20 million expansion of the program. In April 1996, the board approved a second round of grants, increasing the number of state coalitions to thirty over a four-year period. There were some differences between this round and the first round. First, while grantees were funded to strengthen statewide coalitions, to foster public awareness efforts to denormalize tobacco use, and to enhance tobacco prevention and treatment capacity, the call for proposals specifically asked applicants to address tobacco policy issues in their state. This change signified that the Foundation's comfort level with advocacy work had increased, and that its overall approach to policy work was maturing. Second, all of the grants awarded under this round—which ranged from $200,000 to $1.5 million—were implementation grants. Finally, and perhaps most significantly, the program incorporated a "special opportunities fund," with $3 million held in reserve for those times when coalitions needed additional support to respond to unforeseen opportunities. This fund, which was administered by the AMA, allowed for a quicker response than would have been possible at the Foundation.

The next year, 1997, was a turbulent one for tobacco control. The National Cancer Institute announced that the ASSIST program would close in 1999, and that responsibility for funding state tobacco control efforts would be assumed by the CDC. Smoking rates were declining slightly among adults, but remained high among young people. The science of tobacco control was improving the understanding of the problem and its solutions, but it was also making clear that it would be a long time before significant reductions in tobacco-related disease and death occurred. State attorneys general were bringing lawsuits against the tobacco industry requesting damages for the huge costs states incurred to treat sick smokers. At The Robert Wood Johnson Foundation, Michael Beachler, the primary architect of the SmokeLess States program, left the Foundation. Early in 1998 (a year that also saw the signing of the $206 billion Master Settlement Agreement between forty-six states and the tobacco industry), Karen Gerlach, an epidemiologist, became the Foundation's officer responsible for overseeing the program.

With all this turmoil in tobacco control and a new program officer overseeing SmokeLess States, a decision was made to buy some time in order to assess how best to move forward. In order to do that without losing some states whose funding would be ending soon, in July 1998, the Foundation's board authorized $6 million to continue support for the original nine implementation states. Several months later, Kathleen Harty left as the deputy director of the NPO in order to lead the Minnesota foundation created as a result of the state's settlement with the tobacco industry. She was replaced by Donna Grande, who brought years of experience at the national level with ASSIST and at the state level with Arizona's SmokeLess States project. (Grande was named codirector of the national program in 2000.)

In late 1999, Michelle Larkin joined the Foundation from the CDC's Office on Smoking and Health. She worked with other Foundation staff members to conduct a wide-ranging review of SmokeLess States. Foundation staff members spent much of the year talking to the program's national partners (the federal government, the major health voluntary organizations, and other organizations working on tobacco control) and assessing the makeup of the National Program Office and the National Advisory Committee. This review led to a request for what became the program's final renewal, in July 2000. The board authorized $52 million over three years to expand SmokeLess States to all fifty states and the District of Columbia, with a major shift in the direction of the program. The program would now focus solely on advocacy regarding tobacco policy. To highlight the significance of the shift, the tag line of the name was changed from "Statewide Tobacco Prevention and Control" to "National Tobacco Policy Initiative," the National Advisory Committee was restructured, and a new logo was designed.

In this, the final phase of the program, the Foundation required states to concentrate exclusively on advancing policies that would reduce tobacco use. These included increased prices (through excise taxes, for example), comprehensive clean indoor air policies, and expanded public and private insurance coverage of tobacco dependence treatment. Coalitions funded under previous rounds of the SmokeLess States program could apply for implementation grants of up to $1.5 million over three years. States that were not funded previously under the SmokeLess States program could apply for a capacity-building grant, which allowed them time to develop the coalition and its policy action plan. If their capacity-building benchmarks, such as diversifying the coalition's membership, securing matching dollars, and developing a clear and achievable policy action plan, were met, the coalition could then apply for an implementation grant.

In their proposals for an implementation grant, applicants needed to demonstrate an understanding of the policy environment within the state, to provide details of other efforts in the state to reduce tobacco use, and to explain how the Foundation's support would complement those efforts. They had to present a policy plan and show that financial resources from other organizations, including unrestricted funds that could be used for lobbying, would be available. They were also required to address how they would carry out program activities while complying with the Foundation's terms of grant. To build a stronger base of support for the policy efforts that would become the focus of the grant, applicants were required to diversify their coalitions beyond the mainstream organizations, particularly the health voluntaries and the medical societies that had been the mainstays of the program in previous years. The Foundation and NPO staffs believed that broader membership would better reflect the makeup of society as a whole and would allow new organizations to bring their perspectives and their power bases to the issue.

With the new policy focus of SmokeLess States, it became necessary to revisit the membership of the National Advisory Committee, or NAC, which was changed to bring in representatives of new organizations that would be essential partners in getting work done in the states. In addition to representatives from the American Cancer Society, the American Heart Association, and the American Lung Association, the Foundation added to the committee representatives from the federal government's National Institutes of Health and CDC, the American Legacy Foundation, the Tobacco-Control Section of the California Department of Health Services, the Center for Tobacco-Free Kids, and the Asian Pacific Partners for Empowerment and Leadership. Four of the original National Advisory Committee members were also included in the new committee.

Additionally, the role of the NAC changed. In addition to their primary responsibility for reviewing proposals and recommending sites for funding, the committee's members took on additional duties: reviewing benchmarks proposed by the coalitions, conducting site visits with the NPO and Foundation staff members, and providing technical assistance to grantees.

The Foundation received proposals from all fifty states and the District of Columbia, and awarded grants to forty-two states and the District. Some state coalitions, including many that had been grantees in the program for years, had difficulty adapting to a policy-only approach to reducing tobacco use. Many tried hard to continue their past efforts that were more educational in nature, such as holding health fairs and distributing brochures on the harm caused by tobacco. In a few states, the department of health had grown to rely on the coalition to implement many of its programs and to garner public support for tobacco-prevention and cessation initiatives. While this remained an important role in the field, it was no longer the objective of the Foundation-funded program. Moreover, the close connection between the coalitions and the state health departments complicated the coalitions' ability to do policy-related work, since governmental agencies are prohibited from taking an active role in making policy.

To assist the coalitions' transformation from programmatic to policy activities, the NPO staff made site visits and provided technical assistance on developing policy action plans. Where intensive assistance was needed, the NPO staff made referrals to experts on particular issues, such as strategic planning, grassroots organizing, working with diverse populations, fundraising, and media relations. Despite the intensive technical assistance provided by the NPO, some coalitions were unable to make the transition to a policy focus, and did not meet their benchmarks. The more hands-on approach to technical assistance created some apprehension among the NPO staff and many of the states, especially those that had been in the program from the beginning. As a consequence, there was a high turnover of staff members at the NPO, resulting in a loss of continuity there and some loss of momentum in the states.

Despite the challenges, the state coalitions supported in the last round of SmokeLess States achieved more than had been expected. Although the precise impact of the Foundation's support cannot be determined, more than thirty states raised their cigarette excise taxes, some more than once. In addition, six states—Connecticut, Delaware, Maine, Massachusetts, New York, and Rhode Island—as well as many cities and towns, enacted comprehensive clean indoor air laws that cover all workers, including those in restaurants and bars. The methods employed by the coalitions are illustrated by the examples of New York State and Oregon.

■ Over the years, the New York coalition had developed good rela-tionships with policymakers. When legislators were found to be interested in learning more about clean indoor air, the coalition took the opportu-nity to educate them through nonpartisan research and analysis on the health and economic benefits that California and other smoke-free places were experiencing. This evidence, coupled with results from opinion polls showing public support for clean indoor air, helped to spur action. The coalition knew that lobbying assistance would be needed, so it used matching dollars (that is, money not from The Robert Wood Johnson Foundation) and hired some experienced lobbyists. A bill eliminating smoking in public places throughout the state was introduced and passed.

■ The coalition in Oregon had two primary goals: to expand Ore-gon's smoke-free workplace law and to increase access to smoking-cessa-tion services. It also had the secondary goal of building momentum for a cigarette tax increase. Because Oregon was experiencing substantial bud-get deficits, the coalition felt that the time was right to pursue its sec-ondary goal, so it focused its attention on increasing the tax on cigarettes. It conducted an extensive public education campaign. It also raised over $240,000 in non–Robert Wood Johnson Foundation funds to lobby legislators about the allocation of the tax dollars and to support the measure on the ballot. In September 2002, Oregonians approved a ballot measure raising the cigarette excise tax by sixty cents.

In 2003, Risa Lavizzo-Mourey became the Foundation's fourth president. She took over at a time when less money was available for programs and the Foundation was reconsidering its priorities. Through a process in which the Foundation developed a more focused grantmaking approach, tobacco was selected as one of eight areas that would continue to receive funds in the future. The amount of support would be, however, much less than it had been in the past, and in July 2003 it became clear that the SmokeLess States program would not be renewed. In August 2003, the Foundation notified the AMA that the NPO would close in May 2004, although some grants under the program would continue beyond that date. Soon thereafter, this was made public in a letter co-signed by Lavizzo-Mourey and Michael Maves, the chief executive officer of the AMA. Many of the grantees reacted with great disappointment to the announcement and expressed concern for the future of tobacco-control advocacy in their states. Since the announcement, Foundation staff members have been working to determine the most strategic ways to maintain the policy infrastructure that had been supported by the SmokeLess States program. As of mid-2004, that future is still being planned.

—ᴠᴠ— Concluding Thoughts

As the SmokeLess States program draws to a close, we, the program officers at The Robert Wood Johnson Foundation overseeing it, would like to offer some reflections. The Foundation invested more than $99 million in SmokeLess States during the ten years the program was active. This represents over 20 percent of the $420 million the Foundation invested in tobacco control since 1992. These are remarkable resources and represent a long-term commitment for a private foundation. The magnitude of the problem of tobacco use, however, required large financial and human resources over an extended period of time, and our concern is that even these resources might not have been sufficient to make the gains permanent.

Those of us at The Robert Wood Johnson Foundation who were responsible for the SmokeLess States program should have acted sooner and more aggressively in developing comprehensive approaches to sustaining the efforts of the states. The program relied heavily on the three major health voluntary organizations—the American Cancer Society, the American Heart Association, and the American Lung Association—to provide financial support, particularly funds that could be used to support lobbying efforts the Foundation could not and did not support. In retrospect, we should have encouraged the coalitions to diversify their funding sources earlier so that the burden didn't fall so heavily on these organizations. When an economic downturn hit in 2000–2001, their ability to support these efforts declined significantly. We should also have helped the coalitions reach out to local funding sources. Although the NPO did provide guidance about fundraising to the coalitions in the final years of the program, it may have been too late to keep some of the coalitions afloat financially.

A second thought is that the efforts to diversify the coalitions were not as successful as we would have hoped. When the program was expanded in 2000, we expressly requested that states diversify their coalition membership. Yet even when diversification became one of the benchmarks for progress, many states made only minimal efforts to expand. They explained that diversification took too much time and too many resources, thus diminishing what was available to do the work of the coalition. We were naïve. We did not realize how difficult diversification was going to be for most of the coalitions. We do not believe that most of them understood why we were adamant about diversification—that the movement will not survive if it does not grow to represent the population of the state. Although the NPO made a heroic effort, and many states made significant progress, there is still much work to be done to truly diversify the movement. We believe it is critical for this work to continue.

A third thought is that clear benchmarks and the ability to measure progress are critical. Benchmarks allowed the NPO and the grantees to work together to make adjustments along the way. As important as it is to know if progress was being made, measuring coalitions' performance against the benchmarks met with strong resistance, especially among those who had not been previously monitored in such a manner. We believe that utilizing benchmarks and offering technical support to help coalitions meet them were well worth the effort, and improved the performance of the coalitions. In many instances, the coalitions were successful in meeting the benchmarks, but some were unable to meet them, and we had to make tough decisions about whether to continue supporting their efforts.

A fourth observation is that advocacy, though not a strategy employed frequently by foundations, can be an effective way to improve the health of the public. Yet advocacy work is messy, and overseeing it is time-intensive. This kind of grantmaking requires astute legal assistance and strong leadership. Fortunately, SmokeLess States was able to benefit from both. The program forged new ground at the Foundation, but, despite its success, there has been minimal uptake of advocacy as a tool in our grantmaking arsenal. Perhaps we should do more to interest other foundations in this approach to addressing important social issues.

Finally, we learned how vital it is to recognize the contribution of grantees and their staffs. Each year of the program, an annual meeting of the coalitions was held in the state that had experienced the greatest policy victory in the previous year. Originally, the meeting was held in the state that increased its tobacco tax the most, but the final annual meeting was held in Delaware to recognize the coalition and the state for enacting the most comprehensive clean indoor air law in the country. These events not only helped the grantees see one another on their home turf instead of at a conference center but they also allowed us to recognize the grantees for the hard work they had done. In hindsight, we should have celebrated their achievements more than just annually.

Despite these challenges, we believe that the program was a success. It exceeded our policy advocacy expectations and provided important insights into how to do this work more effectively. Many of these coalitions continue to expand their membership, moving toward a more inclusive power base. Most of the SmokeLess States coalitions have expressed intentions to continue to work on tobacco-policy advocacy post Smoke-Less States and are engaged in securing resources to support this work.

The demonstration program that was SmokeLess States ended in 2004. The AMA, the National Program Office staff, and the grantees showed great commitment and dedication to this important work. The health of all Americans has been improved by their efforts. Time will tell what the lasting impact will be.

Notes

1. Hughes, R. "Adopting the Substance Abuse Goal: A Story of Philanthropic Decision Making." *To Improve Health and Health Care 1998–1999: The Robert Wood Johnson Foundation Anthology.* San Francisco: Jossey-Bass, 1999.
2. Schapiro, R. "A Conversation with Steven A. Schroeder." *To Improve Health and Health Care, Vol. VI: The Robert Wood Johnson Foundation Anthology.* San Francisco: Jossey-Bass, 2003.
3. Chapter One in this volume.
4. Gutman, M. A., Altman, D. G., and Rabin, R. L. "Tobacco Policy Research." *To Improve Health and Health Care 1998–1999: The Robert Wood Johnson Foundation Anthology.* San Francisco: Jossey-Bass, 1999.

Reducing Youth Drinking

The "A Matter of Degree" and "Reducing Underage Drinking Through Coalitions" Programs

Susan G. Parker

Editors' Introduction

Drinking among young Americans is a serious health problem. Yet the familiar refrains of "Boys will be boys" and "We did it when we were young" make it difficult to focus attention on behavior that is a central factor in automobile fatalities, rape, unsafe sex, and suicide. In many ways, alcohol is the hidden health issue of the younger generation, obscured by the publicity given to tobacco, teenage pregnancy, and illegal drugs. The difficulty of bringing the issue to the public's attention is compounded by a number of other factors: this country's history of prohibition, which makes it easy to label those concerned with youth drinking as neoprohibitionists; the strength of the beer and alcohol industry; and the evidence that wine, taken in moderation by adults, is beneficial to health.

There have, however, been efforts—some of them successful—to raise public consciousness. Mothers Against Drunk Driving, spearheaded by mothers whose children were killed or injured by drunk drivers, had a stunning success in changing public attitudes toward drinking and driving. Along with Remove Intoxicated Drivers and Students Against Drunk Driving, Mothers Against Drunk

Driving can take credit for legislation lowering the legal drinking age to eighteen and the legal limit of alcohol in the blood to .08 percent.

It was in this complex environment that The Robert Wood Johnson Foundation began, in the early 1990s, to address the harm caused by underage drinking, first by financing a survey of alcohol use and abuse in colleges and then by funding a series of programs aimed at reducing drinking from elementary school age through university level. In this chapter, Susan Parker, a freelance journalist specializing in health, religion, and business, examines the Foundation's programs to curtail drinking among the young, particularly its two flagship programs: A Matter of Degree, and Reducing Underage Drinking Through Coalitions. A Matter of Degree has provided funding to ten universities to develop programs that would make the environment on campus and in surrounding communities less hospitable to underage drinking and binge drinking. Reducing Underage Drinking Through Coalitions has supported state-based coalitions of citizens working on youth leadership programs, public awareness campaigns, and innovative uses of public policy to reduce underage drinking. In this chapter, Parker looks at the history and the rationale of these programs, how they operate in practice, and the early findings from evaluations. She concludes by drawing lessons based on site visits and interviews with national experts, program evaluators, and participants in the programs.

~~~~ I t was Thursday night, the beginning of the weekend for many college students. Corey Domingue, a nineteen-year-old chemical engineering major at Louisiana State University, or LSU, and his friends headed to a nearby grocery store, where they bought hard liquor. When they arrived back at their off-campus apartment, Domingue was interested in partying. He opened a bottle of rum and began to drink rum and coke steadily. At around 12:30 A.M., he began to feel sick and started throwing up. A friend dragged him into the bathroom, where he fell asleep. At 4:30 A.M., a friend returned to the bathroom and found that Domingue was having trouble breathing. He called 911. Paramedics arrived and tried to revive Domingue, to no avail. He was rushed to a hospital, but workers there were unsuccessful as well. Domingue died of acute alcohol poisoning. He had consumed about a fifth of rum in just a few hours. His blood alcohol level was .43—five times the .08 legal limit for driving. He died in spite of having received warnings about the dangers of alcohol from his father, who is a recovering alcoholic. Corey Domingue himself had warned his younger sister not to drink.

Domingue was a former high school honor student and football star who was the first in his family to attend college. His death, in October 2003, was a senseless end to a promising young life. It was also a blow to LSU. The university has fought its image as a party school, and in recent years had been part of a national demonstration program, A Matter of Degree, funded by The Robert Wood Johnson Foundation, to reduce binge drinking and the harm associated with heavy drinking among college students. LSU decided to join the program in part because of the negative nationwide publicity it had received over the alcohol-poisoning death in 1997 of twenty-year-old Benjamin Wynne, who died after consuming an estimated twenty-four drinks in celebration of a bid to his fraternity, Sigma Alpha Epsilon.

At the time of Domingue's death, LSU Chancellor Mark Emmert told reporters, "We have spent so much time and so much energy trying to educate our students about the risks of binge drinking, and it was particularly painful to lose someone in such an obviously preventable way. . . . We're seeing more and more students already engaged in binge drinking. They're not learning this in college. In many ways, they're already binge drinkers by the time they get here."[1]

Drinking is the hidden problem of young people, obscured by the sight of kids smoking cigarettes and ads that target illegal drug use among adolescents. But alcohol is the most frequently used drug among young Americans. In 2003, some 75 percent of high school students had experimented with alcohol, compared to 58 percent who had tried cigarettes and 53 percent who had tried any illegal drug (including marijuana and cocaine).[2]

The consequences of alcohol use among underage young people are stark:

- Motor vehicle crashes are the leading cause of death for young people aged fifteen to twenty, and more than one-third of those fatalities involve alcohol. In 2000, alcohol-related fatality rates were nearly twice as high for eighteen-, nineteen-, and twenty-year-olds as for people aged twenty-one and older.[3]

- Alcohol is a central factor in most college rapes. About one in twenty women reported being raped in college and nearly three-quarters of those rapes (72 percent) happened when the victims were so intoxicated that they were unable to consent or refuse. [4]

- Alcohol has been associated with the early initiation of sexual activity and risky sexual behavior that places young people at risk for sexually transmitted diseases, HIV infection, and unplanned pregnancy.[5]

- Among college students, almost half of the frequent drinkers reported five or more binge drinking–related problems, such as blackouts, fights, and missed classes.[6]

- The suicide rate among young people is increasing at an alarming rate. Alcohol use among adolescents has been associated with considering, planning, attempting, and completing suicide. In one study, 37 percent of eighth-grade females who drank heavily reported attempted suicide, compared with 11 percent who did not drink.[7]

- The earlier children start drinking, the more likely they are to be harmed by its use. Those who start drinking before age fourteen are twelve times more likely to be injured while under the influence of alcohol sometime in their life than those who start later.[8]

Binge drinking—defined by Harvard School of Public Health researchers as five or more drinks in a row for men and four or more for women—is a matter of particular concern. Students who binge drink frequently tend to get into fights, damage property, engage in unprotected sex, become victims of sexual assault, miss classes, and fall behind in schoolwork. Students who do not drink heavily but attend colleges where a lot of drinking takes place report that their property has been damaged by drunk students; that they have been pushed, hit, or insulted, or have experienced an unwanted sexual advance; and have had to cope with the aftereffects of someone else's drinking, such as cleaning up a roommate's vomit. Despite an overall decline in drinking in the United States, there has been no decrease in binge drinking on college campuses since 1993, when the Harvard School of Public Health College Alcohol Study first measured it nationally. "On many campuses, drinking behavior that would elsewhere be classified as alcohol abuse may be socially acceptable, or even socially attractive, despite its documented implication in automobile crashes, other injury, violence, suicide, and high-risk sexual behavior," Harvard researcher Henry Wechsler and his colleagues wrote in the *Journal of the American Medical Association.*[9]

—ᨆ— **Why the Importance of Addressing Underage Drinking Is Not Appreciated**

Even though underage drinking, particularly binge drinking, has serious health consequences to the drinker, his or her roommates and neighbors, and the community, these consequences are not widely appreciated. One reason is that excessive drinking is sometimes seen as a normal part of late adolescence or, perhaps, a rite of passage. This "boys-will-be-boys" attitude is pervasive. One college administrator noted that when his school decided to participate in the A Matter of Degree program, alumni complained that the tradition was being sucked out of fraternities—that students should be left alone to have fun. Alums vilified college officials as trying to cut the spontaneity out of the place and hurting the campus climate. Students donned T-shirts saying that the program "sucks." Parents worried that if the school succeeded in reducing drinking, their kids might turn to drugs.

At the University of Colorado at Boulder, students rioted over the program. At the University of Nebraska–Lincoln, Kevin Koss ran for student body president on the platform of getting rid of NU Directions, the school's A Matter of Degree program. "I like to party and drink and I don't think it should be other people's job to legislate and regulate how we do it," said Koss, a junior who plays for the school's rugby team. Koss lost the election.

As these comments imply, those who seek to curtail drinking among young people are accused by some of being neoprohibitionists. John Doyle, executive director of the American Beverage Institute and a frequent critic of Robert Wood Johnson Foundation–funded programs, wrote, "This movement is eerily similar to the movement that gave us Prohibition. Like the early 20th century movement, it is well-organized, it is self-righteous, and it has sympathetic ears in the media. And considering that nearly all of its supporters seem to be bankrolled in some way by the $8 billion Robert Wood Johnson Foundation, it's even better funded than its pre-Jazz Age forbear."[10] Dan Mindus of The Center for Consumer Freedom, a coalition representing restaurants and the food and alcohol industry, wrote that The Robert Wood Johnson Foundation has turned alcohol providers into "public enemy number one, burdening them with restrictions and taxes to make their business as difficult and complex as possible."[11]

It is probably not surprising that members of the alcohol industry have attacked these programs, since cutting down on the drinking of college students and other young people threatens their bottom line—as it does the bottom line of manufacturers, wholesalers, retailers (liquor stores and others who sell alcohol), bars, and restaurants. Together they make up a formidable opposition at local, state, and national levels.

The alcohol industry has been a daunting opponent at several Robert Wood Johnson Foundation–funded program sites. At Florida State University, for example, the local beer industry used its money and clout to derail a coalition to curb student alcohol abuse. Anheuser-Busch and others in the alcohol industry successfully challenged the coalition's plan to end underage access to bars, increase penalties for serving underage drinking, restrict alcohol marketing, and eliminate low-priced drink specials.[12]

Finally, unlike tobacco and illegal drugs, alcohol is not necessarily dangerous in limited amounts. In fact, the benefit to health of a daily glass or two of wine has received much publicity. Thus, it is the abuse, not the use, of alcohol that is dangerous. In addition, for minors, any consumption of alcohol is, of course, illegal.

—⟍⟍— The Robert Wood Johnson Foundation's Programs to Reduce Youth Drinking

In 1990, at the behest of The Robert Wood Johnson Foundation's new president, Steven Schroeder, the staff and the board of trustees re-thought the Foundation's broad goals. As a result, in 1991 the Foundation adopted as one of its goals reducing the harm caused by substance abuse. The following year, Henry Wechsler, of Harvard School of Public Health, came to the Foundation with a proposal. He had conducted small studies at New England colleges that showed an alarming percentage of college students were drinking heavily and harming themselves and others. He wanted to conduct a national study to see if these problems occurred at campuses around the country. At about the same time, a poll of college presidents named drinking as the number-one problem on campuses.[13]

As a result, the Foundation commissioned the College Alcohol Study, the first nationally representative survey of college drinking. Wechsler and his colleagues surveyed more than 17,000 students at 140 colleges about their drinking habits. They found that nearly half of the college students (44 percent) were binge drinkers and almost a fifth (19 percent) were frequent bingers. The study found that one of three binge-drinking students was already a binge drinker the year before college.[14]

The findings from the survey—which became the first in a series of Robert Wood Johnson Foundation–funded College Alcohol Studies carried out by Wechsler and his colleagues—generated nationwide media coverage. The studies were the first to document the extent of heavy drinking in colleges across the country. According to Wechsler, the findings influenced the National Institute on Alcohol Abuse and Alcoholism and the Centers for Disease Control and Prevention to give attention to this issue and the Surgeon General to make a reduction of heavy drinking in college a national goal.

In response to the College Alcohol Study findings and other data, in 1996 the Foundation funded two new national programs to address drinking by young people. The first was A Matter of Degree, an $8.6 million program designed to reduce binge drinking among college students by fostering collaboration between universities and the communities where they are situated. The program, which is scheduled to run through 2007, targets universities with a high percentage of students who are heavy drinkers. The second, Reducing Underage Drinking Through Coalitions, an eight-year, $10.2 million initiative, addresses the problem of drinking among even younger people, those in junior high and high school. The American Medical Association serves as the national program office for both programs.

Experts in the field of preventing alcohol abuse among young people tend to favor either an educational or an environmental approach. The former focuses on teaching young people, often through peer education, about the potential harm of alcohol use to themselves and others. If people have the facts about the problems that alcohol can cause, advocates of the educational approach say, then they may be willing to change their behavior. This approach is a comfortable one for educational institutions, including colleges, which believe in the power of education. It is also touted by the alcohol industry, which stresses individual responsibility.

A variation of the educational approach is a social-norms strategy. According to William DeJong, a professor of social and behavioral sciences at Boston University School of Public Health and a leading researcher on this approach, this strategy assumes that students have inaccurate and in-flated perceptions of how much drinking is going on. Social-norms campaigns give students information about the realities of drinking, thereby reducing the influence of peer pressure to drink and reinforcing the behavior of most students, who purportedly drink either moderately or not at all.[15]

Both A Matter of Degree and Reducing Underage Drinking Through Coalitions largely employ an environmental approach. While education remains an important part of the programs, they primarily look to change the factors that influence young people to drink, such as easy access to alcohol and the failure to penalize illegal drinking. Both programs have relied on the establishment of local coalitions. "Conceptually, each program was based on the understanding that a public health approach had to be at the core," said Marilyn Aguirre-Molina, a former Robert Wood Johnson Foundation program officer who helped design the programs. "These are community issues and community problems that have community roots. You can't do this in isolation." According to Aguirre-Molina, research shows that educational programs, at least the traditional individually oriented ones, make little or no impact on drinking behavior. She noted that the Foundation hoped that the new programs would provide models of approaches that might work to reduce underage and binge drinking.

In designing these programs, staff members built on the Foundation's previous experience, especially with tobacco-control initiatives that focused on changing environmental factors (by enforcing laws prohibiting sales to minors, banning smoking in public places, and raising tobacco taxes) and anti–substance abuse initiatives spearheaded by community-based coalitions.[16, 17, 18]

A Matter of Degree and Reducing Underage Drinking Through Coalitions are the largest and most visible components of a more wide-ranging Foundation strategy to reduce young people's drinking. The College Alcohol Study and A Matter of Degree focus on college students. The Center for College Health and Safety, also funded by the Foundation, uses the results from A Matter of Degree to create prevention projects at other colleges and universities. Reducing Underage Drinking Through Coalitions concentrates largely on junior high and high school students. Another program, Leadership to Keep Children Alcohol Free, a coalition of thirty-four governors' spouses and about thirty public and private organizations that the Foundation funds jointly with the National Institute on Alcohol Abuse and Alcoholism, looks to curb drinking among even younger children—those ages nine to fifteen. The Foundation also provides grants for a biannual national alcohol policy conference, where results and lessons learned from Foundation-funded programs are shared with policymakers, opinion leaders, and experts in the field. Another program, The Center on Alcohol Marketing and Youth, funded jointly with The Pew Charitable Trusts, monitors and analyzes the alcohol industry's advertising practices targeted at young people.

—w— A Matter of Degree

In A Matter of Degree, colleges with high rates of binge drinking were given the chance to apply for grants of up to $700,000. The schools would form partnerships with their local communities to address alcohol abuse. The program also funded a media campaign that was aimed at deglamorizing student binge drinking. Between 1997 and 1999, grants were awarded to the University of Colorado at Boulder and the city of Boulder; the University of Delaware and the city of Newark, Delaware; Florida State University and the city of Tallahassee; Georgia Institute of Technology and the city of Atlanta; the University of Iowa and the city of Iowa City; Lehigh University and the city of Bethlehem, Pennsylvania; Louisiana State University and the city of Baton Rouge; the University of Nebraska–Lincoln and the city of Lincoln; the University of Vermont and the city of Burlington; and the University of Wisconsin–Madison and the city of Madison.

The universities and communities engaged in a wide variety of activities, among them working toward these ends:

- Eliminating alcohol-industry sponsorship of athletics and other campus social events
- Eliminating the sale of alcohol during sporting events, limiting tailgate parties to pregame only, creating alcohol-

free tailgate zones, and restricting alcohol sales at concerts and other on-campus events

- Establishing higher standards for Greek organizations, including academic achievement, community service, and adherence to campus and community alcohol policies

- Adopting policies requiring that parents be notified if their son or daughter violated campus alcohol policies or was arrested for an alcohol violation off campus

- Addressing loud house parties and the disruption they created for residents of the community

- Educating, in conjunction with area high schools, prospective students about the university's alcohol policies

- Creating alcohol-free alternative social activities for students and expanding substance-free housing options

The University of Nebraska's NU Directions

NU Directions, the project at the University of Nebraska's Lincoln campus, illustrates the range of activities taking place on one campus and in the surrounding community as well as the difficulty of trying to change deeply rooted social norms of heavy drinking in college.

Lincoln is in the middle of farmland, where, even though the university has a world-class music program and the city boasts a thriving arts community, the University of Nebraska Cornhuskers football team dominates conversation. The NU Directions coalition consists of more than seventy members, including university staff members, students, the Lincoln police chief, neighborhood activists, bar owners, and members of local nonprofit alcohol-prevention organizations, such as the city's detoxification center. The coalition is headed by James Griesen, vice chancellor for student affairs at the University of Nebraska-Lincoln, and Tom Casady, Lincoln's chief of police.

School and city officials knew that they had a major drinking problem to address. The College Alcohol Study had revealed that 62 percent of the students were binge drinkers. In Lincoln, liquor licenses were easy and cheap to come by, with more than 400 licenses registered in a city of

232,000 residents and 22,500 students. Students could choose from about fifty bars within walking distance of campus. When the Cornhuskers played at home, the city transformed itself into one big tailgate party. The university, which was a dry campus, had begun to crack down on parties at fraternity houses, but many students simply moved them off campus. In 1997, the year the program began, city police received 133 citizen complaints about parties at off-campus residences within a mile of the university. City police felt that they had little support from the community or the university in breaking up these parties, according to police chief Casady. "For ten years, we abandoned doing anything about drinking parties other than try and keep the cruisers right side up," Casady said.

NU Directions started with several advantages. The university had a long history of cordial relationships with the community. The original project director, Linda Major, was a long-time community organizer whose contacts ran deep into Lincoln. Once the grant from The Robert Wood Johnson Foundation was approved, the coalition met for a year and created a strategic plan of thirteen goals and sixty objectives. It spent the next four years putting the plan into effect. The coalition worked in four broad areas described below, with varying degrees of success in each:

Social Environment

The coalition sought to provide alternatives for students who relied on heavy drinking as their social outlet. It sponsored events that proved popular on campus, including a homecoming party featuring a well-known band that attracted hundreds of students, and a Back to School Bash that included free pancakes at midnight, sumo wrestling, and dancing. The coalition also created a Nutodo.com Web site that provided information about Lincoln restaurants, theaters, nightclubs, recreation centers, sports arenas, and events. Vendors listed had to sign a "Responsible Hospitality Agreement," in which they promised to work to prevent sales of alcohol to minors by training their staff in responsible hospitality practices, such as not serving intoxicated patrons and avoiding promotions that encourage high-risk drinking, such as offering cheap pitchers of beer.

Kevin Koss, who lost the election for student body president on a platform of eliminating NU Directions, was later appointed to the coalition by the incoming president, who felt that the group needed more of the perspective of the students that the project targeted. Koss's opinion of the coalition has shifted, at least somewhat. "They have been pushing nonalcohol things at night, which is good because it makes the community more interesting," Koss said. "They bring in bands and movies. There are nice things you can do at the student union. That way, a lot of people are not getting bombed. A lot of people show up having had a few drinks but at least they are not drinking while they are there."

Neighborhood Relations

The coalition instituted a "party patrol" of off-duty Lincoln police officers, some of whom work undercover, to find large parties with underage drinkers. The police issued citations to students and others for violations such as selling alcohol without a license, procuring alcohol for a minor, and maintaining a disorderly house. The coalition began the party patrol after its data showed that most students did their heavy drinking at off-campus parties. In one weekend, the party patrol issued more than 134 citations—about half to University of Nebraska students. The police followed up each weekend sweep with a press conference with details on the citations, including the names of those who received citations.

Not surprisingly, this turned out to be one of the least popular activities of the coalition among University of Nebraska–Lincoln students. Emmy Thomas, an editorial writer for the student paper wrote of the party patrols, "Yes, just as they've done each of the past three years I've been a student here, Lincoln's police force has again pledged to 'crack down' on 'wild parties.' And they are keeping that promise this time around, despite what seems to be a complete absence of anything wild on this campus. . . . In other words, the cops in this town have decided to sniff out any group of more than five people listening to anything other than classical music at a decibel level over 10."[19]

On-Campus Policy and Enforcement

The University of Nebraska also stepped up enforcement of state law and its policies against underage drinking on campus. Campus police began writing more citations for students caught with alcohol. The citation, called Minors in Possession, carries a $124 fine, a trip before the school's judicial affairs board, and mandatory attendance at an educational program on alcohol use and abuse. "We have a philosophy that if you make a conscious decision to violate policy and laws, it should be a conscious decision to accept the consequences," said Owen Yardley, the campus chief of police.

Yardley also began cracking down on tailgating before Cornhuskers games. About 80,000 people descend on Lincoln for the games, many of whom get ready to cheer for the Cornhuskers by drinking in the parking lots. It sent a mixed message to students that while they were being targeted for drinking, all sorts of alcohol-fueled rowdiness and damage was overlooked on game day, Yardley said. Campus officials sent out letters to all season ticket holders that alcohol was not allowed on university property. According to Yardley, the enforcement has made alcohol consumption less visible during game day. Additionally, for the first time, fraternities violating the university's policy on alcohol lost their privilege to have freshmen—the lifeblood of any fraternity—live in the fraternity house.

Education and Information

One element of the Nebraska program was a "social norms" campaign that aimed at correcting misperceptions among students that all of their fellow students were drinking heavily. The coalition put out pamphlets and other material stating, among other things, that 71 percent of students have zero to four drinks when they go out drinking. Another educational activity took aim at twenty-first-birthday bar "crawls," in which students go from bar to bar, sometimes consuming ten or twenty drinks or more. An ad campaign called Adults Don't Crawl pointed out that most students don't participate in these birthday crawls.

The social-norms approach was controversial among students, researchers, and community members. The student body president, Kyle Arganbright, called it "condescending." James Baird, a coalition member who runs Cornhusker Place, Inc., a detox and alcohol rehabilitation facility in Lincoln, said the campaign irked him for another reason. "It sent a mixed message to the community," said Baird, a former assistant chief of police in Lincoln. "As you go around the community, the public schools, and the courts, it's not OK to drink if you're under twenty-one. Young high school kids interacting with friends at the university see billboards that say 70 percent of people drink four or fewer drinks. They see the message as it's OK to drink."

NU Directions and the Bottom Line

The coalition also attempted, with no success, to limit the number of liquor licenses, to institute mandatory server training, and to reduce certain kinds of marketing, such as the promotion of cheap drink specials. The lack of success is typical of moves by coalitions that could affect the bottom line of businesses. "We can stop one high-risk promotion and there will be another one behind it," said Tom Workman, NU Directions' assistant director for information strategies.

Matt Vrzal, a former player for the Cornhuskers football team, who now owns several bars on O Street catering to University of Nebraska students and is a member of the NU Directions coalition, offers a unique perspective on the tensions and the promise of A Matter of Degree. As a college student, the 330-pound former center frequented the bars using fake IDs, and admits to downing more than thirty shots on his twenty-first birthday, which sent him to the hospital. Now, he said, he watches out for students who drink too much in his bars, limiting service and even paying for taxi rides home.

Vrzal supports the work of the coalition and similar programs. "What a message to send to parents," he said. "This university cares enough about your kids to keep them safe. They don't want them to misuse alcohol, and they don't want them in harm's way." He has noticed a difference in the students who come to his bars. "When the program first started, the kids thought it was a big joke, just another group telling them what to do," Vrzal said. "But NU Directions has done a nice job in distributing the research to the kids. Recently there was this one kid who was taking his friend out for his twenty-first birthday. He said, 'We know what's going on, he's only on one shot an hour. NU Directions said this and that.'"

Yet Vrzal is also critical of the coalition for being out of touch. When he was in college, Vrzal said, "kids took the bars for what they were, places to have fun, not get falling-down drunk and have fights in the street. Now the people in authority positions at NU Directions think it's a debacle down here. . . . They think that O Street and the bar owners are just a bunch of raging alcoholics and people puking in the streets. In reality, they're a bunch of social drinkers having a good time."

The Nebraska project leadership can point to some accomplishments. Data from the Nebraska site shows a decrease in binge drinking rates, from 62 percent in 1997 to 47 percent in 2003. There were also fewer problems experienced by students who drink. Students who reported engaging in unplanned sex declined from 32 percent to 20 percent, and students who reported being insulted or humiliated by another student who was drunk dropped from 43 percent to 24 percent.[20]

Louisiana State University

At Louisiana State University, vice chancellor Neil Mathews says that the university has come a long way since the highly publicized death in 1997 of Benjamin Wynne during pledge week. He said that since A Matter of Degree began there, the university has set up substance-free residence halls, cracked down on the long-standing tradition of bringing alcohol into the football stadium, and tightened enforcement for fraternities violating alcohol policies, including removing some of them from campus. He pointed out that the October 2003 death of Corey Domingue led to the discovery of a false ID ring, which in turn led to felony charges against several students who allegedly sold the IDs. As a result, the LSU Campus-Community Coalition for Change, as LSU's A Matter of Degree program is called, successfully advocated for increased penalties for the production and use of false IDs and for the vendors who sell or distribute alcohol to underage students. Still, Domingue's death, in the face of all of that the university has done to change the environment and attitudes about binge drinking, points to the limits of these programs in the face of such an intractable problem.

Preliminary Evaluation Results

Harvard's Henry Wechsler, who is the principal investigator of the evaluation of A Matter of Degree, said that overall the program was "working at a modest level. Our expectations always were that you're not going to make a major change overnight." Early results from the evaluation did not find significant changes in drinking habits, including changes in the rates of binge drinking, for the ten schools in the program when measured against the schools used for comparison purposes. However, the results also indicated that the schools most fully implementing the program model of environmental change showed declines in alcohol consumption, alcohol-related harm, and secondhand effects. Schools that employed fewer environmental measures and less program implementation showed no such declines.[21] "This tells us that the original design of the program and its rationale—to change the upstream determinants of heavy and harmful drinking—was well conceived," notes Elissa Weitzman, also from the Harvard School of Public Health, who is the co-principal investigator and the director of the Matter of Degree evaluation.

—ɯ— Reducing Underage Drinking Through Coalitions

Reducing Underage Drinking Through Coalitions addresses the problem of drinking among younger students—those in junior high and high school. It was born in part out of the recognition that for many adolescents, drinking starts much sooner than the day they set foot on a college campus. The program provides grants to statewide coalitions that could include law enforcement, youth organizations, the faith community, governmental agencies, alcohol prevention organizations, civic organizations, and businesses. The Robert Wood Johnson Foundation required each program to have four elements: (1) youth leadership development, (2) coalition development, (3) alcohol policy development, and (4) a public awareness campaign. It funded coalitions in Connecticut, Georgia, Indiana, Louisiana, Minnesota, Missouri, North Carolina, Oregon, Pennsylvania, Puerto Rico, Texas, and Washington, D.C. The various coalitions sought to

- Ensure by working with law enforcement agencies that store clerks and alcohol servers do not provide alcohol to minors
- Reduce the availability of alcohol at sporting and community events

- Initiate compliance "stings" of merchants who sell alcohol to minors
- Establish statewide hotlines to report underage drinking and outlets selling alcohol to minors
- Create a statewide keg registration law, which ensures that keg purchasers are held responsible if minors are served
- Tighten ID checks, train alcohol beverage servers, and reduce the use of special pricing that encourages overconsumption
- Train youth leaders, who serve as media spokespersons and testify before state legislatures about the harm of underage drinking
- Enact ordinances to increase the distance of billboards advertising alcohol from schools, churches, and rehabilitation centers

A Variety of Approaches

The Reducing Underage Drinking coalitions spent much of their time in efforts to educate legislators about the problem of youth drinking and ways that state policies could reduce the problem. These efforts were often made more difficult by the fact that many legislators received substantial campaign contributions from the alcohol industry. To counteract the influence of the powerful alcohol industry, coalitions employed a variety of tactics to bring the issues to the attention of the public. For example, they mobilized constituents, organized demonstrations, held press conferences, and fed information to the media.

Some coalitions used a divide-and-conquer approach. The Minnesota Join Together Coalition to Reduce Underage Drinking, for example, found ways to work with some alcohol industry groups while fighting others. The Minnesota Grocers Association wanted grocery stores to be allowed to sell wine, a move opposed by the coalition as providing another easy way for young people to get alcohol. The coalition found an ally in the retail liquor industry, which did not want competition from grocery stores, according to Jeff Nachbar, the Minnesota project director. Coalition members agreed to do public education that would help the liquor industry defeat the proposal. In return, the liquor industry worked with the coalition on keg registration—a mandatory tagging system that enables police to trace the purchaser of a keg of beer—something many liquor store owners had opposed as being onerous. The keg registration effort was successful.

Several coalitions focused on eliminating alcohol advertising in certain publications, billboards, and other venues that young people would see. This has proved to be a difficult task. In Texas, the coalition spent three years in an ultimately successful effort to eliminate alcohol and tobacco advertising from the Texas Parks & Wildlife Department's hunting and fishing guide. Anyone who is older than eight must take a quiz on the guide to get a fishing or hunting license. About 40 percent of the ads were alcohol or tobacco promotions. In 1999, Jim Haire, who is an avid outdoorsman and works at a sporting-goods store, noticed that the guidebook was filled with alcohol and tobacco ads. Worried about the effect of these ads on children, including his own, he went to Texans Standing Tall, the state's Reducing Underage Drinking Through Coalitions site, to talk about his concerns.

Coalition members took up the issue, and in their research learned that the state legislature would be reviewing the Texas Parks & Wildlife Department to determine whether it should be reauthorized—a process that all state agencies must undergo every ten years or so. They saw the reauthorization as their opening to push for the elimination of the advertising. Using Texas's open records law, coalition members learned that Anheuser-Busch, which produces Budweiser beer, had contributed millions of dollars to the Texas Parks & Wildlife Department and had created a Parks and Wildlife Foundation of Texas, which played a major role in the production of the hunting and fishing guide. Coalition members pointed out that this collaboration generated conflicts of interest, among them that the department in charge of reducing alcohol-related boating accidents was accepting alcohol advertisements. Coalition staff and members testified that the department's authorization should be renewed, provided that the department be prohibited from accepting alcohol and tobacco ads. It won a partial victory when the reauthorization specified that the Parks & Wildlife Department could no longer carry tobacco ads and that it create guidelines for appropriate advertising of alcohol.

For the next two years, coalition members hounded the department to create those guidelines and to prohibit alcohol advertising, according to Ellen Ward, executive director of Texans Standing Tall. It took until 2001 for the department to issue the guidelines, which prohibited the department from accepting ads for tobacco or alcohol products. While Ward is pleased with the results, she said that since the guidelines went into effect Anheuser-Busch has found another venue in which to advertise: the Texas Parks & Wildlife magazine now carries a full-page advertisement from Budweiser, which it had not done in the past. Despite the apparent inconsistency with the department's own code, coalition members have not yet been able to persuade it to get rid of the ads in a publication that is distributed to middle school and high school libraries.

The Connecticut Coalition to Stop Underage Drinking is located in one of the country's most affluent states, where many adolescents have plenty of money and parents supply alcohol to their underage children. Children in Connecticut start drinking, on average, at age eleven—the youngest age of any state in the country. According to the project director, Gary Najarian, the rates of drinking among young people are almost 30 percent higher than the national average.

The Connecticut coalition, like others, worked to change alcohol policy at the state level, with varying success. According to Najarian, the coalition gathered several state organizations that had not worked together on underage drinking before and brought attention to the issue through press conferences and news coverage. That public education work contributed to three of the coalition's objectives becoming state law: (1) keg registration, (2) underage participation in compliance checks (sending young people to liquor stores to try to buy alcohol), and (3) banning alcohol sales at convenience store drive-up windows.

Early Assessment of Results

Alexander Wagenaar and his colleagues at the University of Minnesota are evaluating the Reducing Underage Drinking Through Coalitions program. In the first phase of their evaluation, they compared public opinion, coalition formation and activities, and state-level alcohol legislation in the coalition states and in the rest of the country. Preliminary results indicate that few states—whether they had a Reducing Underage Drinking coalition or not—passed laws aimed at reducing young people's access to alcohol. The evaluators and the site directors pointed out that the evaluation did not capture all activity on the local level, such as ordinances that change penalties for sales to minors or alter local enforcement procedures. The preliminary findings indicated that the coalitions focused most of their policy work on commercial access policies (compliance checks, false identification, minors not allowed in bars, outlet density, and server training) and the least on pricing (excise taxes, licensing fees, and price discounting).

—w— Observations

A Matter of Degree and Reducing Underage Drinking Through Coalitions are emblematic of a new approach to battling the problems of adolescents' drinking and hurting themselves and others. Rather than focus just on educating individuals, these programs seek to change the environment in which alcohol is depicted as sexy, glamorous, hip, and easily available. It is an approach that relies on coalitions of sometimes uneasy allies. These programs, which have been in effect for only about eight years, are trying to shift mores and norms that have existed for decades. It is still too early too tell whether they will have an effect. However, participants, national experts, and evaluators made several observations about what can be learned to date from the programs.

■ *There were unrealistic expectations in some quarters about what could be accomplished in a short time.* According to Joan Hollendonner, a former senior communications officer at The Robert Wood Johnson Foundation who oversaw its programs to reduce college high-risk drinking and underage drinking, there were unrealistic expectations on the parts of some Foundation staff and board members, reporters, and members of the public about what the programs could accomplish in the original grant periods. (A Matter of Degree was initially funded for four years and Reducing Underage Drinking Through Coalitions for five years.) She stated:

To expect to see significant drops in the actual rates of college binge drinking or underage drinking in those timeframes was naïve. The programs used a new approach to change social norms, policies, and practices. It was anticipated that in turn drinking rates would be lowered and harm reduced. First, however, the sites had to plan their efforts and learn, educate, and create buy-in for this very different (environmental) approach to prevention. Then you are talking about changing an extraordinarily deep-rooted norm in this country that tolerates youth drinking and overcoming resistance to shifts in policies and practices. Just for people to grasp the environmental approach was difficult. The entire task at hand was enormously challenging, and it required time and patience. Fortunately the programs were renewed.

■ *The complicated interactions that lead many adolescents and college students to drink or drink to excess cannot be addressed through one program or narrow approach.* The environmental approach has been shown to work in areas such as drinking and driving, but has not been fully tested in an area as complex as underage drinking. Educational programs may still have their place, and there may be other approaches not yet discovered. "We're starting to see over time that there is a cumulative effect of the interacting of many factors," said Richard Yoast, of the American Medical Association, who is the national director of A Matter of Degree and Reducing Underage Drinking Through Coalitions. "There is not going to be one thing that will make the change. It's not like we can suddenly introduce a vaccine."

■ *The programs take on powerful, entrenched economic interests that are difficult to dislodge.* Both of these programs challenge the economic interests of the alcohol industry, from manufacturers to retailers to bar owners. It is always a tough fight to make changes that threaten an industry's bottom line.

■ *It is difficult to break out of the educational approach and embrace the environmental one.* Taking an environmental approach promised and proved to be difficult for universities and prevention agencies, both of which were steeped in the world of education, not advocacy. "It's much easier to think about gathering up kids and talking to them about the evils of drinking than talking to adults and telling them they are doing things that make the environment easier for kids to drink," said Eileen Harwood, an evaluator at the University of Minnesota of the Reducing Underage Drinking Through Coalitions program.

■ *Coalitions provide a promising way to tackle long-standing social problems, but it is also difficult for them to take tough stands.* In many cases, the programs brought together groups with diverse interests that had never collaborated before, and it was hard to persuade them to take controversial stands. Broad-based coalitions are more inclined to work in areas where reaching consensus is comparatively easy, such as providing alternative activities for students, than in more difficult areas, such as raising taxes on liquor and enforcing underage drinking laws.

■ *It is difficult to mobilize a movement around the harmful effects of alcohol on others as tobacco control advocates have done around cigarettes.* It is still hard for many people to see heavy drinking by young adults as anything other than an inevitable rite of passage into adulthood. "We have yet to effectively promote a movement around second-hand effects of alcohol," said Harvard's Elissa Weitzman. "It's hard to argue that a single cigarette is good for you. But a glass of wine for most people is not a problem. Alcohol occupies a unique place. It's not altogether bad. But that makes it hard for people to come up with a position on it or find themselves willing to change important aspects of its availability."

While alcohol plays a complex role in our society, young people need to know that their community has set a standard for behavior around drinking, several project directors said. Evaluators and project directors said that adolescents and college students saw no adverse consequences for their excessive drinking and so had no reason to stop. John Bishop, the project director for Building Responsibility, the A Matter of Degree site at the University of Delaware, conducted focus groups with students about drinking. He found that at the beginning of the project "students really didn't believe that the university was serious about enforcing alcohol regulations." Now the university has set up a "three strikes and you're out" policy for alcohol violations that include parental notification, monetary fines, and possible expulsion.

Focusing on the harms that alcohol use causes others may prove effective in the long run just as it has for the tobacco control movement.

One of the biggest changes that program directors note is an awareness of the effects of drinking on others, through increased fights, sexual assaults, and disturbances. "Initially, the main focus of A Matter of Degree was on reducing the binge-drinking rate," the American Medical Association's Richard Yoast said. "That's not something we're shying away from, but most people are less concerned about how much is drunk than what happens when too much is drunk. If you tell students we are going to reduce the amount of alcohol you are drinking, many will have no interest in that. If we talk about the problems they and their peers are having, most students—drinkers and non-drinkers alike—are very interested. They are the ones who are subjected to fights, disruptions, and vomit. They are the ones who are sexually harassed."

Notes

1. "LSU Tries to Recover from Latest Tragedy." Associated Press, October 21, 2003.
2. CDC. "Despite Improvements, Many High School Students Still Engaging in Risky Health Behaviors." Press release, May 20, 2004 (www.cdc.gov/od/oc/media/pressrel/r040520b.htm); CDC. "Tobacco Use by Young People." Tobacco Fact Sheet (wwwwcdc.gov/HealthyYouth/tobacco/facts.htm); CDC. "Youth Risk Behavior Surveillance—United States—2003." *Morbidity and Mortality Weekly Report,* May 21, 2004.
3. National Highway Transportation Highway Safety Administration. *2000 Youth Fatal Crash and Alcohol Facts.* Washington, D.C.: National Highway Transportation Highway Safety Administration, 2001.
4. Mohler, K. M., Dowdall, G. W., Koss, M. "Correlates of Rape while Intoxicated in a National Sample of College Women." *Journal of Studies on Alcohol,* 2004, 65(1), 37–45.
5. Kaiser Family Foundation. *Survey Snapshot: Substance Use and Risky Sexual Behavior, Attitudes and Practices Among Adolescents and Young Adults.* Menlo Park: Calif.: The Henry J. Kaiser Foundation, 2002.

6. Wechsler, H., Lee, J., Kuo, M., Nelson, T., and Lee, H. "Trends in College Binge Drinking During a Period of Increased Prevention Efforts: Findings from 4 Harvard School of Public Health College Alcohol Study Surveys: 1993–2001." *Journal of American College Health,* 2002, *50*(5), 203–217.

7. Substance Abuse and Mental Health Services Administration. *Summary Findings from the 1998 National Household Survey on Drug Abuse.* Rockville, Md.: U.S. Department of Health and Human Services, 1999.

8. Hingson, R. W., Heeren, T., Jamaka, A., et. al. "Age of Drinking Onset and Unintentional Injury Involvement after Drinking." *Journal of the American Medical Association,* 2002, *284,* 1527–1533.

9. Wechsler, H., Davenport, A., Dowdell, G., Moeykens, B., and Castillo, S. "Health and Behavioral Consequences of Binge Drinking in College: A National Survey of Students at 140 Campuses." *Journal of the American Medical Association,* 1994, *272,* 1672–1677.

10. Doyle, J. "Prohibition, Drip by Drip." *California Wine and Food,* 2003.

11. Mindus, D. "Behind the Neo-Prohibition Campaign: The Robert Wood Johnson Foundation." (www.consumerfreedom.com). April 30, 2003.

12. Gruley, B. "How One University Stumbled in Its Attack on Alcohol Abuse." *Wall Street Journal,* October 14, 2003.

13. The Carnegie Foundation for the Advancement of Teaching. *Campus Life: In Search of Community.* Princeton, N.J.: Princeton, University Press, 1990.

14. Wechsler, H., Davenport A., Dowdall, G., Moeykens, B., and Castillo, S. "Health and Behavioral Consequences of Binge Drinking in College." *Journal of the American Medical Association,* 1994, *272* (21) 1672–1677.

15. "An Interview with William DeLong." *The Report on Social Norms.* (www.socialnormslink.com/default.asp). September 2003. DeJong directs the U.S. Department of Education's Higher Education Center for Alcohol and Other Drug Prevention (which The Robert Wood Johnson Foundation partially funds), which helps colleges

develop social norms campaigns. DeJong and his colleagues are carrying out a randomized trial involving thirty-two campuses, with sixteen randomly assigned to do a social norms marketing campaign and sixteen assigned to a no-campaign control group.

16. Chapter One in this volume.
17. Wielawski, I. "The Fighting Back Program." *To Improve Health and Health Care, Vol. VII: The Robert Wood Johnson Foundation Anthology.* San Francisco: Jossey-Bass, 2003.
18. Chapter Two in this volume.
19. Thomas, E. "Drinking Age Should Drop by Three Years." *Daily Nebraskan,* September 5, 2001.
20. Harvard College Alcohol Study, 2003. Boston, Mass.: Harvard School of Public Health.
21. Weitzman, E. R., Nelson, T. F., Lee, H., Wechsler, H. "Reducing Drinking and Related Harms in College: Evaluation of the 'A Matter of Degree' Program." *American Journal of Preventive Medicine.* Forthcoming.

The Robert Wood Johnson Foundation's Commitment to Nursing

Carolyn Newbergh

Editors' Introduction

With the nation facing a severe nursing shortage whose causes are more deeply rooted than those of any previous shortage, The Robert Wood Johnson Foundation responded, in 2002, by designating nursing as one of its eight targeted areas and by making a decade-long commitment to strengthening the nursing profession. While this is the first time the Foundation has singled out nursing as an explicit grantmaking priority, it is not the Foundation's first venture into nursing. In fact, since its inception as a national philanthropy, The Robert Wood Johnson Foundation has invested more than $140 million in nursing programs.

It is natural that a foundation whose mission is improving health and health care would give such attention to nursing. The nation's 2.7 million registered nurses make up the single largest part of the health care workforce and are, in many ways, the backbone of the health care system. Strengthening nursing at all levels allows the Foundation to advance two of its long-standing interests: increasing access to high-quality care and improving the health care workforce.

Previous volumes of *The Robert Wood Johnson Foundation Anthology* series have featured chapters on specific nursing programs.[1] In this chapter, Carolyn Newbergh, a freelance journalist and frequent contributor to the series, reviews the entire range of the Foundation's nursing programs, beginning with early initiatives to build the new profession of nurse practitioner, continuing with its programs to improve academic nursing and strengthen hospital nursing, and concluding with its current programs to develop the leadership skills of high-level nurses and to transform the working conditions of hospital nurses.

Newbergh finds that the Foundation's relatively consistent commitment to nursing has helped strengthen the profession, but also that the erratic nature of the Foundation's entry into and exit from specific programs in the past led to missed opportunities and tarnishing of its image within academic nursing. Nonetheless, the wide range of approaches adopted by the Foundation to advance nursing—fellowships, bolstering of academic departments, demonstration projects, research, publicity, support of professional organizations—provides a good illustration of how philanthropy can, over many years, help build a field.

---

1. Keenan, T. "Support of Nurse Practitioners and Physician Assistants." *To Improve Health and Health Care 1998–1999: The Robert Wood Johnson Foundation Anthology.* San Francisco: Jossey-Bass, 1999; Rundall, T. G., Starkweather, D. B., Norrish, B. "The Strengthening Hospital Nursing Program." *To Improve Health and Health Care 1998–1999: The Robert Wood Johnson Foundation Anthology.* San Francisco: Jossey-Bass, 1999; Bronner, E. "The Teaching Nursing Home Program." *To Improve Health and Health Care, Vol. VII: The Robert Wood Johnson Foundation Anthology.* San Francisco: Jossey-Bass, 2004.

—ɯ— T̲he nation's 1.3 million hospital nurses are in critical condition. Beset with heavy caseloads of sicker patients than they've ever cared for before, they work in jobs that earn them little respect, offer limited autonomy, and hold out slim possibility for advancement or professional reward. Worst of all, nurses feel frustrated that they cannot always give patients the kind of quality care they deserve; giving such care is, after all, the reason that they became nurses in the first place. As a result, many nurses—particularly hospital nurses—are leaving the profession, while the number of those entering it has slowed to a trickle. This situation has created a nationwide nursing shortage that is broader and more complex than any that has existed before.[1]

The roots of America's nursing shortage can be traced to the mid-nineteenth century, when altruistic women toiled in the homes of people who could afford them, and then in charity hospitals for the poor—always there to serve physicians who valued them for their manual labor, rather than for any critical thinking they could bring to bear. They were exploited during their early apprenticeship training in hospitals, where they cooked and nursed for up to sixteen hours a day and were paid only in room and board. After two years of this, they received a diploma.[2]

Nursing schools were first accredited in the 1930s, and educational standards for nurses were raised. Gradually, hospitals began to be staffed by graduate nurses rather than student nurses, but the nurses still labored for long hours with no independence, little assistance, and low pay. The Second World War brought on a nursing shortage as women left the hospital wards to fill society's wartime needs. By the 1950s, with an explosion in new medical technologies and a great increase in the number of hospitals after passage of the Hill-Burton Act in 1948, nurse training became too expensive for hospitals and had begun to move largely into associate degree programs at two-year community colleges. By then, there were three paths to becoming a registered nurse—a two-year hospital diploma, a two-year associate degree, and a four-year baccalaureate degree. Although each route involved different amounts of education and clinical training, most hospitals made no distinction in work or pay among the three—and they still don't. Over time, physicians transferred many responsibilities, such as administering intravenous medications, taking blood pressure, and inserting catheters, to nurses—but still for no extra pay or increase in status.

—⚉— The Current Nursing Shortage

Poor working conditions, low pay, little possibility of advancement, and increased career opportunities for women in other professions have led to today's severe shortage of nurses. One study put job dissatisfaction at four times as high for nurses as for all other kinds of workers.[3] It also found that one in five nurses was expected to resign within the coming year. Another study showed that the nation's hospitals were short 126,000 nurses in 2002 and would fall behind by 400,000 by 2020.[4]

Nursing shortages have occurred periodically in the past, of course, but the current shortage has some unique structural features that make it more serious than previous ones. "The issues that are problematic in nursing are the same that have always been there," said Linda Aiken, a professor at the University of Pennsylvania School of Nursing, who, as a vice president of The Robert Wood Johnson Foundation, helped develop its nursing programs from 1974 to 1987. The current shortage is more worrisome than past shortages, Aiken noted, "because of changes in utilization patterns in hospitals, the shortening length of stays, and the move to outpatient surgery. People who are in the beds are much sicker and require more intensive nursing care."

The nation's demographics threaten to make this nursing shortage far worse still. The baby boom generation, 78 million strong, will start reaching age sixty-five in 2011. And as more Americans reach sixty-five, and live well into their seventies, eighties, and nineties, many will be beset with multiple chronic illnesses and will require complex care. As the population is aging, so is the nursing workforce. The average age of today's hospital nurse is slightly over forty-three, the oldest it's ever been.[5] In fact, more nurses are over fifty than under thirty-five, the age group that one would expect to provide the largest number of nurses. Because the work is so physically strenuous, large numbers of older nurses can be expected to retire soon.

Complicating the picture further, too little fresh blood is flowing in. For the last twenty years, far fewer women have ventured into nursing as more potentially satisfying career options have become open to them. Those who do choose to become nurses frequently feel overwhelmed and unprepared for work on the hospital floor—an estimated 35 to 55 percent of brand new nurses leave within the first to third years of work, according to Geraldine Bednash, executive director of the American Association of Colleges of Nursing. Meanwhile, at a time when new nurses are desperately needed, the nation's nursing schools are actually turning prospective students away because of lack of space to teach them.

There is one bright spot in this otherwise gloomy picture: a 2003 study found that the number of nurses in the workforce grew during 2002. Nearly all of this gain, however, was attributed to the use of foreign-born nurses and to married women over fifty returning to work during the economic downturn. As the economy improves, fewer retired nurses will have an economic incentive to return to their former profession.[6]

—∿— The Robert Wood Johnson Foundation Support of the Nursing Profession

Recognizing that nursing is in crisis, various professional organizations, government agencies, and philanthropies have produced analytical reports and have come up with plans to tackle the problem. The Robert Wood Johnson Foundation has weighed in too. As part of a broader strategy to improve the quality of the nation's health care, the Foundation, in 2002, designated nursing as one of its eight priority areas and launched a major new initiative to overhaul hospital nursing.

The Foundation is no newcomer to nursing, however. Its efforts to bolster the profession have been ongoing, though intermittent, throughout its history (see Figure 4.1). Indeed, the Foundation has been a major philanthropic funder of initiatives to strengthen the field of nursing, along with the W.K. Kellogg Foundation and, to a lesser degree, the Helene Fuld Health Trust and the John A. Hartford, Independence, Jewish Healthcare, and Josiah Macy, Jr. foundations.

Since becoming a national philanthropy in 1972, The Robert Wood Johnson Foundation has invested about $140 million in nursing programs

Figure 4.1   National Nursing Programs

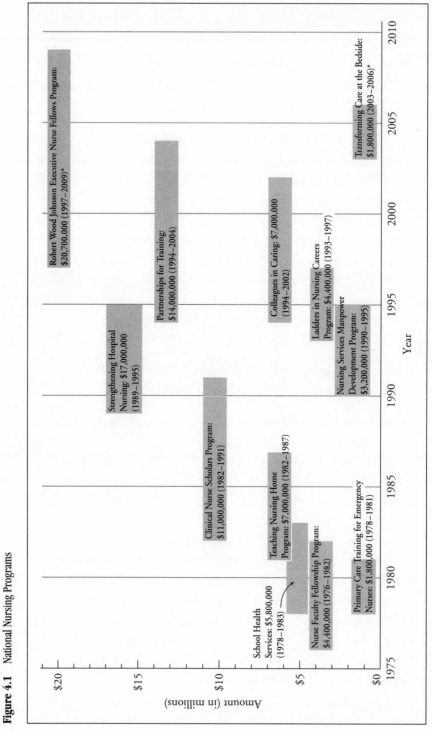

*May be renewed or expanded

of varying magnitude and lifespan. Its initial nursing grants in the 1970s and the early 1980s were devoted to increasing access to primary care outside of hospitals through the enhanced training of nurses to be nurse practitioners. Its grants supporting the education of nurse practitioners are regarded as critical to legitimizing nurse practitioners as health care professionals. The Foundation then branched out and supported efforts to strengthen nursing within institutions, largely by improving patient care and nurses' work environment within hospitals and by encouraging minorities to enter nursing.

—〰— The 1970s and Early 1980s: Strengthening Nurse Practitioners and Nursing Education

Ask virtually anyone who is knowledgeable about nursing whether The Robert Wood Johnson Foundation has made any lasting contributions to the profession and the nearly universal response is that its work was instrumental in developing nurse practitioners as providers of primary care outside the hospital. "I think it would be safe to say the Foundation had a major role in the development and mainstreaming of nurse practitioners," Linda Aiken said. "In addition to giving money for programs, it gave legitimacy to the idea, which was very important."

Early Nurse Practitioner Programs

When The Robert Wood Johnson Foundation began promoting nurse practitioners in 1973, the field was relatively new and controversial. Although a few physicians had provided their nurses with training that enabled them to deliver care beyond their current scope of practice, and some schools had begun certifying these new midlevel practitioners, the field was nascent, with just 4,000 nurse practitioners nationwide. There are more than 100,000 today. "The nurse practitioner concept then was disliked by nursing deans, who thought we were taking their nurses and making doctors or doctor extenders out of them," said Terrance Keenan, who, as a Foundation vice president, shepherded most of the Foundation's early nursing efforts. "Doctors were suspicious that we were giving nurses authority to do clinical interventions that were beyond their education."

At the time, the nation was experiencing a physician shortage in rural and low-income urban areas—a shortage brought on by the retirement of older physicians who had been practicing alone. Meanwhile, about 700,000 nurses—most of them not practicing, some working in physicians' offices—were viewed as an untapped resource. The theory was that with some additional education in such subjects as anatomy, microbiology, pharmacology, and the signs and symptoms of diseases, nurses could become a new type of midlevel health professional trained to diagnose and treat common illnesses and manage stable chronic conditions. This could be achieved for far less investment than the six years or more of education and training required for physicians. The nurses in turn would develop their skills, work mostly independently with backup from doctors, and increase their earnings. The Foundation embraced the use of nurse practitioners as an opportunity to meet its goal of improving access to primary care in underserved areas.

Its first foray into the field was to support nurse practitioner–based community health service networks in urban and rural areas.[7] Notable among these demonstration projects, which generally took place between 1973 and 1978, were these:

- At the University of California, Davis, the new Department of Family Practice trained family nurse practitioners working in a network of doctor-nurse teams. These teams provided care in rural sites that ranged from Pacific coast fishing villages to distant mountain locations.

- The Utah Valley Hospital, in Provo, put together a network of clinics to serve rural residents, many of whom would otherwise have had to travel 200 miles or more to reach the nearest doctor. The hospital's emergency room physicians trained the nurse practitioners, who saw patients in their communities. The doctors, available twenty-four hours a day for emergency backup, would fly to a given area in small planes twice each week to treat patients needing more attention.

- The Tuskegee Institute in Tuskegee, Alabama, trained a nurse practitioner and sent her and a lab technician in a

van to rural sites located in three counties. The van was
equipped with advanced communications technology that
enabled the nurse practitioner to talk by telephone with
physicians at the hospital.

- The Frontier Nursing Service, in Hyden, Kentucky, is
storied for having had the first training program for nurse
midwives. Based in rural clinics, the nurse midwives would
reach their clientele on horseback. The Foundation helped
the Frontier Nursing Service develop a program to train the
nurse midwives as family nurse practitioners as well.

The results of these early demonstration projects convinced the Foundation that nurse practitioners could help expand access to quality primary care. It then funded programs that extended the work of nurse practitioners to two other areas in need of primary health care providers: public schools and hospital emergency rooms.

Starting in 1978, the five-year School Health Services Program brought nurse practitioners into the elementary schools of thirty-six urban school districts serving 150,000 low-income children in four states. Regular school nurses often couldn't handle the volume and the complex needs of these children, who had no other health care providers. The nurse practitioners examined the children, managed illnesses and medications, provided immunizations, and developed care plans for them. However, after Robert Wood Johnson Foundation support ended, the schools found it difficult to find funding from other sources.[8]

Another trouble spot was the rural hospital emergency room. With fewer physicians available there, nurses were inundated with patients complaining of rashes, sore throats, and other nonemergency maladies. What these patients needed was routine primary care, not expensive and limited emergency care. In response, the Foundation funded the $1.8 million Program to Equip Emergency Nurses with Primary Care Skills. This program, which ran from 1978 to 1981, prepared emergency room nurses to become nurse practitioners and provide the primary care needed by many emergency room patients. Six university-affiliated hospitals gave rigorous primary care training to nurses from small hospitals in each region. Again, when support from The Robert Wood Johnson Foundation ended, the program's leaders couldn't find enough other financial support to continue it.

The difficulty that the School Health Services Program and the Program to Equip Emergency Nurses with Primary Care Skills encountered raising money led the Foundation's staff to think about how best to support the nurse practitioner field. The approach of boosting the field through demonstration projects had been tried. Now the thinking was that nurse practitioner training needed solid footing within higher education—namely, in primary care master's degree programs within nursing schools.

Grants that the Foundation had awarded to graduate nurse practitioner programs at six universities had helped to establish the profession within academia, but they also revealed that nurse practitioner education was in need of qualified teachers. The Foundation then initiated the $4.4 million Nurse Faculty Fellowships in Primary Care, which ran from 1976 to 1982. It aimed at creating an elite core of leaders in nurse practitioner education who would return to teaching after completing their fellowships, and help establish master's degree programs. Ninety-nine nurse fellows were trained at four nursing schools and became pioneers for nurse practitioner education around the nation. "The impact those ninety-nine people have had is significant," said Geraldine Bednash, the executive director of the American Association of Colleges of Nursing and herself one of the fellows. "Nurse Faculty Fellowships in Primary Care was an important element in sending out people committed to the development of nurse practitioners."

The fellowship program was not renewed in 1982, as questions arose about whether there would actually be a need for more nurse practitioners and Congress was preparing to support nurse practitioner education. Many within and outside the Foundation questioned the wisdom of not continuing the program, but its legacy continues. "We now have this wonderful group of nursing leaders," Bednash said. "They have assured that nurse practitioner education will remain as an important part of nursing education."

The Teaching Nursing Home Program

From 1982 to 1987, the Foundation found another setting in which nurses and nurse practitioners could extend primary care to an underserved population. It established the $7 million Teaching Nursing Home

Program, which had the grand ambition of creating nursing homes where nursing students, many of them enrolled in nurse practitioner programs, would receive on-the-job training—just as medical residents received on-the-job training in teaching hospitals. The eleven demonstration sites attempted to improve the care of the residents through the affiliation of nursing schools with nursing homes. It was hoped that this approach would also trim the nursing home's costs by reducing the length of residents' stay in the home or in the hospital.[9]

The program improved outcomes for the nursing home residents (an evaluation found that it had reduced hospitalizations and showed "some evidence of higher quality care" in comparison to other nursing homes[10]), but it never took off as a model nationally. It did have some lasting effects, however: more nurses and nurse practitioners work in nursing homes today, geriatrics is now a standard component of nursing education, and the program's evaluation played a role in shaping the way care of the elderly is assessed.

The Clinical Nurse Scholars Program

It was an unusual twentieth reunion that took place in San Diego in November 2003, commemorating the start of the Clinical Nurse Scholars Program. The alumni of this program, which produced just sixty-two graduates, included deans and assistant deans of nursing schools, nurses who held distinguished chairs in nursing schools, and senior faculty members in nursing around the nation.

Also among them were nurses who had become researchers noted for such work as infant sucking and feeding, postpartum depression and the immune response, infection control methods, the negative effects of bed rest on pregnant women, cardiovascular nursing, short-term psychotherapy for breast cancer survivors, and a test to measure pain in children.

Twelve years after Clinical Nurse Scholars shut its doors, the fellows still regretted that The Robert Wood Johnson Foundation had discontinued the program that they had found so vital to their careers and to the advancement of nursing education in this country. "All of us said Clinical Nurse Scholars launched us in our careers," said Shannon Perry, who became director of San Francisco State University's School of Nursing.

"We have eminent scholars who are mentoring upcoming scholars; we have deans of schools of nursing with a vision because of some of the things they were exposed to in the Clinical Nurse Scholars Program. We have colleagues around the nation we can call on."

The program began in 1982 as a way to solve a major problem: nursing schools were turning out graduates lacking in practical clinical experience to handle the challenges of the hospital floor. At considerable expense and frustration, hospitals were having to devote time to training these nurses in the basics of hospital care. The nurses themselves started their careers in a sort of culture shock because they weren't prepared, leading many to leave hospital work. The goal was to train outstanding postdoctoral nurse educators in the realities of clinical practice. They, in turn, would lead efforts to infuse nursing education with this knowledge and experience. The new program was modeled on two earlier Foundation programs: the Clinical Scholars Program for physicians and the Nurse Faculty Fellowships in Primary Care.

While praising the quality of the Clinical Nurse Scholars Program, the Foundation truncated it because it was emphasizing research far more than had been intended, and at the expense of clinical teaching expertise. Seven classes of Clinical Nurse Scholars—instead of the intended ten—completed the two years of training, which was held at three universities. The Foundation's president, Leighton Cluff, noted in a 1987 letter to a member of the program's advisory committee that Clinical Nurse Scholars "had assumed the character of a postdoctoral nurse research fellowship in clinical problems, rather than serving as a resource for training a cadre of clinically superior teachers in hospital nursing, as originally intended."

Those involved in the program say that it was the Foundation that missed the mark. It didn't understand that for nurses to gain prominence as leaders, they needed to follow the same path as the nation's most noted doctors—by developing expertise in research. The Clinical Nurse Scholars Program did just that, they said, by teaching its participants how to find sources for research funding, how to go about getting it, and then how to conduct research.

Today the Clinical Nurse Scholars alumnae lament that no other program has taken its place in building the elite nursing faculty of the future.

"What's worrisome is we're getting older and not many of us are left," Perry said. "Some of us were mid-career then, and now we're getting close to retirement. We need to develop a whole group of good scholars again."

—ⱳ— The 1980s and Early 1990s: Addressing the Nursing Shortage

The Strengthening Hospital Nursing Program

By the late 1980s, 80 percent of the nation's hospitals were struggling with nursing shortages: closing beds, canceling elective surgeries, and diverting ambulances to other hospitals. Burned-out nurses were stretched thin and quitting, and nursing school enrollments plummeted. Hospitals lured nurses with signing bonuses and recruited them from the Philippines, England, and other countries.

One of the underlying problems was the working conditions of hospital nurses. Nurses complained that they had little authority to make patient care decisions on their own, and were often treated dismissively by doctors. Although nurses were well paid when they entered the field, their pay never rose much in succeeding years. They spent too much time filling out forms and running around after medications and food—tasks better suited to someone not needed at the bedside.

To address this situation, The Robert Wood Johnson Foundation and The Pew Charitable Trusts sponsored the $26.8 million initiative, Strengthening Hospital Nursing: A Program to Improve Patient Care. At the time, it was the largest investment by philanthropies in a nursing initiative. The Robert Wood Johnson Foundation's share was $17 million. After awarding planning grants to eighty hospitals, the demonstration program set twenty hospitals loose to design changes in hospital systems that would improve patient care by removing the impediments that nurses faced in providing bedside care. The Foundation hoped that by improving the nursing work environment fewer medical errors would be made, patients would have swifter recoveries, money would be saved, and more people would be attracted to nursing and stay with it. Ideally, innovative models would be found that could be reproduced in hospitals around the country.[11]

Strengthening Hospital Nursing, which ran from 1989 to 1995, aimed at changing anything in the hospital work environment that kept nurses from giving their best to patients. The hospitals tried many approaches—including case management teams of physicians, support staff, and nurses that coordinated care; more authority and independence for nurses; new protocols for tasks, including the delegation of some routine tasks to support staff; and a two-year residency program for newly graduated nurses.

At one hospital, for example, a case management team tried to reduce the length of time antibiotics were given intravenously. During the team's daily rounds, the nurse would ask the patient how he or she was feeling. The minute the patient said, "I feel better," the team would make an assessment and if it was appropriate, take the patient off the IV and start oral antibiotics. As a result, the risk of infections from an open line was reduced and a substantial amount of money was saved. Another hospital reduced readmissions of obstetrics patients 75 percent by having nurses teach the women how to care for themselves and their babies before they left the hospital and by sending nurses on home visits afterward.

"So many of the ideas were simple," Barbara Donaho, the program's national program director, said. "This program was about validating instincts about what needed to be done or what people knew would be accomplished if the whole team did it that way. When one unit began to have a success, another unit would do something similar. It infiltrated the entire hospital organization."

During this program, the nursing shortage turned around. Managed care companies pressured hospitals to cut costs, which led hospitals to lay off nurses. Consequently, Strengthening Hospital Nursing seemed to lose its purpose. Moreover, some within the Foundation questioned whether the twin goals of strengthening hospital nursing and improving patient care at the same time were compatible after all. Others faulted the program for allowing hospitals to try so many approaches that it was hard to compare them and choose models to reproduce. When the program came to an end, the Foundation did not renew it.

Nevertheless, many voices praised Strengthening Hospital Nursing. An outside evaluation described changes made by the hospitals as running "deep and wide." It cited a number of accomplishments: "Core patient care processes were redesigned, affecting the practice patterns and the working relationships among many different clinical care providers. In many cases, patient care practice was for the first time standardized." The evaluators added that eight Strengthening Hospital Nursing sites made "lasting improvements in patient care, and in most cases created new models of nursing practice and new relationships among nurses and other providers of care."

The Nursing Services Manpower Development Program

One issue not addressed by the Strengthening Hospital Nursing program was the low participation of minorities in nursing. In the late 1980s, just 8.5 percent of the nation's nurses were minorities. To try to remedy this problem and help ease the nurse staffing shortage, the Foundation mounted its $3.2 million Nursing Services Manpower Development Program from 1990 to 1995.

This relatively small program cast a wide net to see if innovative models could be found for recruiting minorities and individuals who were not traditionally attracted to the field, such as older single parents and men. Through its seven sites, the program provided participants with clinical experiences and other types of assistance that would better prepare them for work in nursing. For example, I'M READY, the project at the University of Illinois at Chicago, reached out to African American and Hispanic students from seventh grade on, giving them information about careers in health care and then supporting them to satisfy the academic requirements for entry into a nursing program. Project Overlap in Indiana helped high school juniors, especially minority students, gain admission to nursing schools, apply for financial aid, and overcome problems such as lack of transportation. The Nurse Recruitment Coalition in Pittsburgh provided minority and nontraditional students with psychosocial support, tutoring, and help with computers and study habits.

Ladders in Nursing Careers

At about the same time, the Foundation was supporting the Ladders in Nursing Careers, or LINC, program in New York City, which helped entry-level and midlevel health care workers in hospitals and nursing homes get the education they needed to enter nursing and advance in the field. During their participation in the program, housekeepers, nurses aides, security guards, and secretaries attended nursing school full-time and worked part-time, while receiving full salary and benefits from their institutions. These employees would not otherwise have been able to attend school. Of the 419 employees in the program, more than two-thirds were minorities and more than 50 percent were single parents. Three-hundred-ninety of them graduated from a nursing program; 90 percent of them passed the state licensing exam.

In light of these positive results, the Foundation funded a $5 million initiative to replicate Ladders in Nursing Careers nationwide. Like the New York program, the national Ladders in Nursing Careers program, which operated from 1993 to 1997, enabled health care workers to go to school full-time and work part-time while continuing on full salary and benefits. The program paid their tuition and related expenses and provided support services, such as one-on-one counseling, review study sessions, and skills enhancement classes. In exchange, these employee-students agreed to give the hospital or other health care organization that sponsored them eighteen months of service for each year they were in the program, up to a maximum of four years.

Like many other Foundation programs in the 1990s, Ladders in Nursing Careers ran into an unexpected roadblock—managed care. With its emphasis on short hospital stays, low reimbursement formulas, and outpatient care, managed care led hospitals to reduce their nursing staffs substantially. As a result, the Ladders in Nursing Careers program was modified in 1995. In addition to training employee-students to enter the nursing field, it prepared them to work in other health care jobs, such as physical therapy and respiratory therapy, where hospitals needed workers. In 1997, when the program ended, 934 employees—nearly 40 percent of them minorities—had participated in it. Of the total, 826 were enrolled in nursing degree programs and 108 in related health fields. An evaluation of the Ladders in Nursing Careers program found that it had achieved its objectives and that "it showed that a project originating in an urban environment can be replicated in other sites, including rural ones."

—〰— The Mid- and Late 1990s: Enhancing the Education of Nurses and Nurse Practitioners

Partnerships for Training

Eleven years after The Robert Wood Johnson Foundation's last foray into nurse practitioner training had ended, it picked up the thread again with a program called Partnerships for Training. This $14 million program, which ran from 1994 through 2004, funded eight regional partnerships in twelve states to expand primary health care to medically underserved urban and rural communities. Developed to address one of the major obstacles faced by prospective nurse practitioner students from underserved areas—the inability to go away to school because of the expense or family obligations—it also tackled a related problem: nurses who left rural areas to get nurse practitioner training rarely returned home. The idea behind the program was that students could be trained in their own communities, where they would be more likely to remain to practice their professions. Thus, rather than have students leave home to become nurse practitioners, physician assistants, and nurse-midwives, Partnerships for Training brought education to them via distance learning technologies. Partnerships were forged between forty-six universities (they provided the academic degree program) and community organizations and leaders (who identified potential students, often helped support them financially, and frequently served as mentors).

It turned out that the thinking behind the program was right. Nearly 90 percent of the 1,200 graduates—most of them trained to be nurse practitioners—remained in their communities. Typical of the graduates is Faye Warren, a nurse for twenty years in Clinton, North Carolina. She worked in her full-time job and cared for her family while studying on-line in the distance learning nurse practitioner program at Duke University. After she graduated, Paul Viser, a physician in her community, hired her to work with him in his practice instead of choosing a physician, as he had done before. "I needed someone who could see patients, and I was looking for a colleague, not an employee," Viser said.

Partnerships for Training had its challenges. For example, much of the original training was done by video teleconferencing; when the technology changed and material could be transmitted more easily and cheaply by the Web, making the transition involved work that had not been anticipated or budgeted. Moreover, some faculty resisted teaching students via long-distance computer technology.

Despite the challenges, those associated with the program have been positive about it. "This 'grow-your-own' model is proving to be one of the most successful ways to date of increasing the number of primary care practitioners in health professional shortage areas," according to a report, *Educating Primary Care Practitioners in Their Home Communities: Partnerships for Training,* produced by the program. Jean Johnson-Pawlson, the program's national director, said that 1,080 additional health care workers staying in their community translated into primary care for 2.5 million people. She noted that even though the Foundation's funding for the program had ended, all the participating schools were continuing to educate students in delivering primary care.

Colleagues in Caring: Regional Collaboratives for Nursing Work Force Development

In 1994, the Foundation authorized Colleagues in Caring: Regional Collaboratives for Nursing Work Force Development, a $7 million, nine-year program aimed at creating workforce development systems with the capacity to meet the shifting demands for nurses. These systems encompassed regional or statewide schools of nursing, nursing employers, professional organizations, and businesses. The program set up twenty regional collaboratives to try to take on the myriad interconnected issues affecting the nursing profession.

The collaboratives collected data on the supply of and demand for nurses in local markets. They mounted initiatives such as nursing recruitment efforts, raised money, planned for long-term needs, and set up a national information-sharing network. Although the collaboratives consisted of people who didn't ordinarily have much to do with one another, "they found many things they could agree on, like setting up long-term planning to meet the needs of the local region from the grassroots up instead of the other way around," said Mary Rapson, director of Colleagues in Caring's national program office at the American Association of Colleges of Nursing. "This was a different approach."

A major accomplishment was setting up systems to address the barriers that different nursing degree programs put up—barriers that discourage nurses from obtaining advanced schooling. Colleagues in Caring worked with the regions and the states to design ways for nurses to return for a higher degree without repeating courses they had already taken, as often occurs. "They opened up a clear and unencumbered educational pathway for nurses to move from diploma training through the baccalaureate without any interruptions," said the Foundation's Terrance Keenan. "A student who graduates with an associate degree from a community college can be admitted to the third year of nursing school at, say, the University of Maryland in Baltimore. That's a big thing. She gets the BSN within eighteen months or two years instead of much longer."

Many sites worked to develop lists of competencies that should be taught at each degree level (hospital diploma, associate degree, baccalaureate degree) so that it would be clear whether nurses had an adequate knowledge base for a particular job. But not much headway was gained in getting hospitals to place nurses in positions commensurate with their education and to compensate them based on the amount of their schooling. "If we don't change the hospital benefit package, we won't get the number of people that we need to go back to school," Rapson said. "There is no incentive for nurses to get higher degrees if they don't get paid better."

An evaluation by The Lewin Group reported that "overall, the program has fostered innovative strategies for addressing nursing workforce development issues. . . . As a result, the program . . . has established a solid foundation and achieved growing recognition both inside and outside the nursing arena."

The Robert Wood Johnson Foundation ended its funding of the Colleagues in Caring program in 2003. Keenan said that the decision not to continue funding "was no disparagement of the program. It was the Foundation's intent to launch a new collaborative effort among all levels of nursing education and nursing care. It was a concept that took hold." According to Rapson, the collaboratives have evolved into "nursing workforce development centers" to continue the work started in the program, and they plan to meet annually to share information. "We started a movement that will go on in some form without us," she said.

—⟋⟍⟍— Today's Nursing Programs

Executive Nurse Fellows

Nurse executives in clinical settings, colleges, and public health are being challenged as never before. Although they have made some strides in reaching management positions in recent years, a glass ceiling allows them to go only so far. Even as the nation wrestles with health care crises, one rarely sees nurses on boards of directors or in leadership positions where they participate in making major decisions.

To bring the most promising nurses into the top tier of health care leadership, the Foundation authorized the Executive Nurse Fellows Program in 1997. It is the Foundation's first nursing fellowship program since Clinical Nurse Scholars ended in 1991. Under the program, each year up to twenty senior nursing executives (from health care services, public health, and nursing education settings) are awarded a three-year fellowship that enables them to receive advanced training in leadership skills. The fellows continue to hold their regular jobs while participating in the program, which takes them away from their home organization for four to six weeks a year.

The program's national program office, located at the Center for the Health Professions of the University of California, San Francisco, evaluates each fellow's leadership skills and then tailors a three-year plan to meet his or her needs. The fellows take seminars and workshops together and do independent studies. Leaders in industries outside of health care share insights about how to anticipate and handle change. A high-level executive, generally from outside of the health care system, serves as a mentor to each fellow. The Robert Wood Johnson Foundation contributes $45,000 toward each fellow's training, while the fellow's employer contributes $30,000 or its equivalent. The employer must also agree to allow time off with pay for the employee to participate in the Executive Nurse Fellows Program.

Marilyn Chow, the program's director and vice president for patient services at Kaiser Permanente's national office in Oakland, California, said she hoped that the training would impart such skills as the ability to inspire, to lead change, and to create strategic vision. "Nurses may not have been given the skills, the mentoring, and the coaching to really be in leadership roles," Chow said. "We're trying to inspire nurse executives. We're taking them out of their narrow clinical focus, helping them to see the bigger picture—how they can transform and lead the kind of delivery systems we will need."

An evaluation of the program by The Lewin Group in 2002 found that the program "fulfills a unique and valuable niche within the nursing arena." Although it was too early to say whether the fellows would become important national nursing leaders, the evaluation noted that they were "gaining a heightened presence beyond their organizations, and, in many cases, beyond the nursing discipline through venues and activities that heighten exposure in ways that may lead to future national leadership roles."

Transformation of Care at the Bedside

In 2002, a Foundation-commissioned study, *Health Care's Human Crisis: The American Nursing Shortage,* laid out the full breadth and depth of the serious nursing shortage of the late 1990s and early 2000s. This shortage, it said, is different from others because it is not just the product of not enough young people entering nursing. What's different is that although the demand for nurses in all health care environments is voracious, nurses, frustrated by their poor working conditions, are exiting in great numbers.

The report did not fall on deaf ears. The next year, The Robert Wood Johnson Foundation made nursing one of eight targeted areas and established a staff team to develop and oversee programs to tackle the hospital nursing shortage. The team is taking on one sizable area of the nursing shortage—improving nurses' work environment so hospitals can attract and hold onto them.

The attention to hospital nursing sprang from the Foundation's renewed emphasis on improving the quality of patient care—and an understanding of how critical nurses are to that goal. "There is a difference in thinking now," said Risa Lavizzo-Mourey, president and chief executive officer of The Robert Wood Johnson Foundation. "We are approaching quality of care from the patient's perspective, and believe that the sorts of issues that create dissatisfaction among hospital patients are also the ones that make the nursing profession dissatisfied with its role. Creating the kind of work environment for nurses that will ensure patient safety and quality of care requires a broad approach and a long-term commitment, entirely consistent with the Foundation's goal to ensure that all Americans have access to quality care at a reasonable cost."

The Foundation has committed $1.8 million through 2006 toward this effort, at which time it will be evaluated for further funding. The nursing team focuses on three target areas: (1) improving the processes and systems that govern nurses' work, (2) promoting the design of hospital buildings that create healing environments for patients and improve worker safety, productivity, and satisfaction, and (3) improving the culture of hospitals. The centerpiece of the nursing team's strategy is an initiative called Transforming Care at the Bedside.

Transforming Care at the Bedside, which has distinct echoes of the earlier Strengthening Hospital Nursing initiative, strives to improve patient care by finding ways to enhance the nursing environment and to allow nurses to concentrate more fully on patient care. "Everything has to do with improving the work environment in hospital settings," said Susan Hassmiller, who leads the Foundation's nursing team. "That's where graduates go when they finish nursing school; that's where a lot of them have their first taste of nursing; and that's what causes them to leave. The work environment is highly unsatisfying for nurses and, in this regard, can and does affect the overall quality of patient care."

The first stage of the Transforming Care initiative was to develop— in collaboration with the Institute for Healthcare Improvement, or IHI, a leader in the field of quality-of-care improvement with headquarters in Boston, and IDEO, a California-based design firm—prototype strategies to improve nurses' working conditions. Strategies focused on the themes of improving safety, eliminating waste, promoting staff vitality, and creating patient-centered environments. Three hospitals, already known to be innovators, were picked to test some of these ideas (such as reducing the redundancy of paperwork), as well as others they generated themselves. The three hospitals then spent ten months, ending in May 2004, testing the strategies in one or two of their medical-surgical nursing units to learn whether rapid testing of small changes at the unit level was feasible.

In the next phase, thirteen leading hospitals were invited to participate in a two-year pilot phase that builds on the work of the three prototype hospitals. Technical assistance from IHI is being provided to help the hospitals make meaningful, sustainable changes. Each participating hospital is required to contribute about $54,000 to IHI to help cover the cost of technical assistance. The Robert Wood Johnson Foundation is supporting all of the initiative's research and development costs, including a two-year evaluation and work with the hospitals' chief financial officers to develop a business case for transforming care at the bedside.

Charging a fee put the Foundation in the unusual position of having to make a business case to sell its own program to potential participants. "The case was fairly simple," Hassmiller said. "If you join us, we'll provide the help needed to help you to keep your patients safe, reduce errors, improve your environments for both patients and staff—and increase your retention of nurses." With an average cost of $40,000 per nurse turnover, the Foundation believes the business case is sufficiently strong to ask hospitals to make the investment. "Without cost data and a business case, it is hard to sway the disbelievers, especially at other hospitals," Hassmiller said. In addition, she noted, the Foundation is making efforts to embed the program within each hospital so that the changes developed under the program will live on after support from The Robert Wood Johnson Foundation ends.

If the pilot phase of the Transforming Care at the Bedside initiative goes well, the Foundation staff hopes to mount a demonstration phase in which many more hospitals will join, but this time they may be asked to adopt one of several specific strategies that are found promising in the pilot phase. In the meantime, the intense interest expressed by other hospitals nationwide has inspired the Institute for Healthcare Strategies and the Foundation to post regular "successful strategies" and other workplace improvement information on their Web sites, make presentations at conferences, and invite other hospitals to meetings.

—⚍— The Foundation's Nursing Initiatives: A Look Back

Reviewing the Foundation's many nursing programs, one is struck by all the stops and starts. The Foundation seemed to hop from one program to another as pressing needs or the current nursing shortage grabbed its attention. Not surprisingly, program participants often say that the Foundation was too hasty in discarding programs for not meeting intended goals when perhaps all they needed was more time. The Clinical Nurse Scholars Program, they note, has had a lasting influence and could have been modified to satisfy the Foundation's misgivings about it. The Nurse Faculty Fellowships in Primary Care, they suggest, was another highly influential program that was halted too early. The questions about the Foundation's unwillingness to stick with its nursing programs extends to the Ladders in Nursing Careers, Colleagues in Caring, and Strengthening Hospital Nursing programs. "The challenge with these efforts is they are about cultural change," Kaiser Permanente's Marilyn Chow said. "It doesn't happen in the time frame that you get funded."

Despite the lack of a coherent strategy in the past,[12] one has to be struck by the long-term commitment the Foundation has made to strengthening the field of nursing. While the Foundation has not devoted to nursing the same kinds of resources that it has to physicians, it has, since its inception as a national philanthropy in 1972, been a strong and relatively consistent supporter of nursing. And it remains so to this day, when, in the context of a serious nursing shortage, it is working to address the fundamental issue of working conditions for hospital nurses.

Notes

1. Berliner, H. S., and Ginzberg, E. "Why This Hospital Nursing Shortage Is Different." *Journal of the American Medical Association,* 2002, *288,* 2742–2744.
2. Hospital nursing programs varied in both quality and duration. Some required as little as one year of training; others required up to three years. On average, students could receive a hospital diploma after two years.
3. Aiken, L., Carke, S. P., Sloane, D. M., Sochalski, J., and Silber, J. H. "Hospital Nurse Staffing and Patient Mortality, Nurse Burnout, and Job Dissatisfaction." *Journal of the American Medical Association,* 2002, *288*(16), 1987–1993.
4. Buerhaus, P. I., Staiger, D. O., and Auerbach, D. I. "Implications of an Aging Registered Nurse Workforce." *Journal of the American Medical Association,* 2002, *283*(22), 2948–2954.
5. *The National Sample Survey of Registered Nurses, 2000.* Washington, D.C: U.S. Department of Health and Human Services Bureau of Health Professions, Division of Nursing.
6. Buerhaus, P. I., Staiger, D. O., and Auerbach, D. I. "Is the Current Shortage of Hospital Nurses Ending?" *Health Affairs,* 2002, *22,* 191–217.
7. Keenan, T. "Support of Nurse Practitioners and Physician Assistants." *To Improve Health and Health Care 1998–1999: The Robert Wood Johnson Foundation Anthology.* San Francisco: Jossey-Bass, 1998.
8. After a three-year lapse, the Foundation continued its support of school-based health services by funding the $20 million School-Based Adolescent Health Care Program between 1987 and 1993

and the $46 million Making the Grade program between 1994 and 2001. The Foundation now funds the Washington, D.C.–based Center for Health and Health Care in Schools to provide technical support to school health programs and to disseminate the idea. Although the concept of school-based health never took off nationally, more than 1,500 elementary and secondary schools (out of a total of 115,000) nationwide currently have health programs staffed by nurses and nurse practitioners. They provide a broad range of services, especially mental health services, to needy children. See Brodeur, P. "School-Based Health Clinics." *To Improve Health and Health Care 2000: The Robert Wood Johnson Foundation Anthology.* San Francisco: Jossey-Bass, 2000.

9. Bronner, E. "The Teaching Nursing Home Program." *To Improve Health and Health Care, Vol. VII: The Robert Wood Johnson Foundation Anthology.* San Francisco: Jossey-Bass, 2003.

10. Shaughnessy, P., and others, "Quality of Care in Teaching Nursing Homes: Findings and Implications." *Health Care Financing Review,* p. 10.

11. See Rundall, T. G., Starkweather, D. B., and Norrish, B. "The Strengthening Hospital Nursing Program." *To Improve Health and Health Care 1998–1999: The Robert Wood Johnson Foundation Anthology.* San Francisco: Jossey-Bass, 1998.

12. Isaacs, S., Sandy, L., and Schroeder, S. "Improving the Health Care Workforce: Perspectives from 24 Years' Experience." *To Improve Health and Health Care 1997: The Robert Wood Johnson Foundation Anthology.* San Francisco: Jossey-Bass, 1997.

5

The Turning Point Initiative

Paul Brodeur

Editors' Introduction

In 1999, The Robert Wood Johnson Foundation formally reorganized its grant-making strategies in a manner that emphasized the distinction between the two elements of its mission: improving health and improving health care. The first element, health, focuses on the nonmedical care aspects of staying healthy, such as behavioral and lifestyle choices, socioeconomic factors, and the public health system. The second element gives attention to the system of medical care that attempts to restore health after illness, injury, or disability occurs.[1]

The 1999 reorganization gave formal recognition to a shift in the Foundation's priorities that had been taking place for a number of years as the Foundation moved toward a more balanced approach to grantmaking between health care and health. In the mid-1980s, the Foundation initiated programs to reduce the harm caused by the use of alcohol, tobacco, and illegal drugs—a focus that accelerated in the 1990s as grantmaking to reduce smoking became a high priority. With the increasing attention being given to health, it became apparent within the Foundation that it had neglected one key component in improving health: the public health system. This was reinforced with the publication of a series of influential books, reports, and articles demonstrating that medical care was responsible for only a small fraction (around 10 percent) of good health[2] and highlighting the weakness of the public health system.[3]

As a result of these internal and external forces, the staff began to consider how the Foundation might play a role in improving the public health. This led, ultimately, to the development and funding of Turning Point, an ambitious initiative designed to transform the nation's public health system. A distinctive feature of the initiative has been the collaboration between The Robert Wood Johnson Foundation, which supports activities at the state level, and the W.K. Kellogg Foundation, which focuses on public health at the county and community levels.[4]

In this chapter, Paul Brodeur, an award-winning health and environmental writer and a veteran author for the *Anthology* series, examines the concept behind and the activities of the Turning Point grantees, highlighting their work in five states. Brodeur also examines the implementation difficulties that the initiative encountered and reviews the reactions—both positive and negative—that Turning Point has evoked in the public health field.

Turning Point was conceived and largely implemented in a pre–September 11th, pre-anthrax world. In some ways, the concerns about bioterrorism and the infusion of federal money for bioterrorism preparedness complicated the initiative, forcing states to deal with terrorism as a transforming event even as they tried to be the forces that transform the public health system. Where public health will end up after Turning Point and post-9/11 is still unclear, but the chapter offers some insights about how the various forces buffeting the public health system are acting and interacting.

---

1. McGinnis, J. M., and Schroeder, S. "Expanding the Focus of The Robert Wood Johnson Foundation: Health and an Equal Partner to Health Care." *To Improve Health and Health Care 2001: The Robert Wood Johnson Foundation Anthology.* San Francisco: Jossey-Bass, 2001.
2. See, for example, McGinnis, J. M., and Foege, W. "Actual Causes of Death in the United States." *Journal of the American Medical Association,* 1993, *270,* 2207–2212; Evans, R., Barer, M., and Marmor, T. *Why Are Some People Healthy and Others Not? The Determinants of the Health of Populations.* New York: Aldine de Gruyter, 1994.

3. Institute of Medicine, *The Future of Public Health.* Washington, D.C.: National Academy Press, 1988.

4. Isaacs, S., and Rodgers, J. "Partnerships Among National Foundations: From Rhetoric to Reality." *To Improve Health and Health Care 2001: The Robert Wood Johnson Foundation.* San Francisco: Jossey-Bass, 2001.

Public health is what we, as a society, do collectively to assure the conditions for people to be healthy.[1]

—w— **I**n 1988, a committee convened by the National Academy of Sciences' Institute of Medicine issued a report finding that the public health of the nation was in an alarming state of disarray. Citing immediate crises, such as the AIDS epidemic, as well as enduring problems such as injuries, chronic illnesses, teenage pregnancy, drug abuse, aging of the general population, and exposure to toxic by-products of the modern economy, this twenty-two-member group—the Committee for the Study of the Future of Public Health—determined that current capabilities for effective public health actions were inadequate, and that "the health of the public is unnecessarily threatened as a result."[2] The committee members also declared that the states "must be the central force in public health," and identified a number of weaknesses in state public health systems—among them lack of funding, the need for partnering with the private sector, and deficiencies in leadership, training, and data gathering and analysis.[3]

Partly in response to the Committee's findings, a working group led by Nancy Kaufman, then a vice president of The Robert Wood Johnson Foundation, and Marilyn Aguirre-Molina, at the time a senior Foundation program officer, began meeting during the early 1990s to devise ways in which the Foundation might help modernize and strengthen state health departments. At about the same time, the W.K. Kellogg Foundation, under the leadership of Gloria Smith, a vice president, had begun work on a plan to revitalize county health departments and community public health. In November 1995, at a roundtable meeting sponsored by the Institute of Medicine, in La Jolla, California, Kaufman and Tom Bruce, a program director at Kellogg, learned for the first time that their respective foundations were working separately toward a common goal. "Tom and I got together that night," Kaufman recalls, "and decided that the only way to proceed was to work together with the understanding that it would take states and communities working together to revitalize the public health system." Since senior executives of the two foundations had already been meeting to explore ways in which they might collaborate, the idea engendered initial enthusiasm among officials of both institutions.

In January 1996, the staff of The Robert Wood Johnson Foundation presented a request to the board of trustees, seeking a two-year $7 million authorization of a new program in which fifteen to twenty states would explore restructuring their public health system, reallocating human and financial resources, developing leadership, increasing the skills of public health officials, expanding the use of technology, improving health surveillance systems and epidemiology, and extending public health partnerships with the private sector. The Kellogg Foundation would collaborate with The Robert Wood Johnson Foundation in this initiative by contributing up to $17 million to support an analogous program at the local level. The $24 million-plus joint venture between the two foundations (which by 2004 had reached a funding level of more than $40 million) represented the largest privately funded effort to strengthen the public health system in the nation's history.[4]

The goal was nothing short of transforming and strengthening the public health infrastructure in the United States. The means of reaching this ambitious goal was the development of collaborative partnerships between public health departments, other state and local health agencies, schools of public health, the business community, health maintenance organizations, hospitals, environmental organizations, and faith-based groups. The timing, as the staff's request to the board pointed out, was urgent: "The window of opportunity presented by the unprecedented changes in the health care environment, the compelling need faced by states to prepare for the increased responsibilities as resources diminish, and the state of the public health infrastructure make this a critical time for intervention."

The new initiative, which was called "Turning Point: Collaborating for a New Century in Public Health," was approved by the board, and in November 1996 a call for letters of intent was sent to potential applicants nationwide. In the call for letters of intent, the Foundation described the essential public health challenges facing the nation as follows: "A study by the Department of Health and Human Services of the ten leading causes of death concluded that only 10 percent of premature deaths are avoidable through improved access to medical care. The remainder were attributed to personal risk behaviors (52%), environmental risks (20%), and human biology (18%). Thus, public health approaches have the potential to prevent the majority of early deaths by targeting factors that contribute to these deaths."

"The response to the call for letters of intent and the subsequent invitation to submit proposals was an avalanche," recalls Bobbie Berkowitz, who directs the Foundation's Turning Point National Program Office at the University of Washington School of Public Health and Community Medicine, in Seattle.[5] "Forty-six states sent proposals to us, and five hundred and twenty-five communities responded with proposals to the Kellogg Foundation. The applications were evaluated for evidence of progressive approaches to the formation of public/private partnerships that would carry out core public health functions and develop new strategies for addressing emerging health challenges. We spent October and November of 1997 sifting through the proposals before winnowing them to twenty-nine, which we sent to the Turning Point National Advisory Committee, whose members winnowed them further to fourteen."

Each of the fourteen states selected—Alaska, Arizona, Illinois, Kansas, Louisiana, Montana, Nebraska, New Hampshire, New Mexico, New York, North Carolina, Oklahoma, Oregon, and Virginia—received a two-year $300,000 grant to develop a plan for modernizing and improving its public health system. At the same time, forty-one communities and counties in the fourteen states received grants of up to $60,000 from the Kellogg Foundation for two to three years of planning and implementation. In order to enhance collaboration, the state partnerships created under The Robert Wood Johnson Foundation grants included the communities funded by the Kellogg Foundation and vice versa. The National Advisory Committee provided overall guidance for the Turning Point initiative, but separate national program offices were designated to manage the grants of each foundation. The Robert Wood Johnson Foundation's grants were administered by a national program office located at the University of Washington's School of Public Health and Community Medicine. The Kellogg Foundation's grants were administered by the National Association of County and City Health Officials, or NACCHO, in Washington, D.C.

—ₘₙ— The Planning Phase

During the planning stage that began in 1998, the initial fourteen grantee states were required to assess public health needs in their state and to submit public health improvement plans with specific goals. (In 1999, The Robert Wood Johnson Foundation awarded planning grants to seven additional states—Colorado, Maine, Minnesota, Missouri, South Carolina, West Virginia, and Wisconsin—bringing the total to twenty-one.) The needs, which varied widely from state to state, were reflected in the range of plans. For example:

- Montana's plan found a need for better training and education of its state and local public health personnel, and called for the establishment of a public health training institute.

- The Turning Point initiative in Louisiana gave priority to expanding access to and quality of health care for people living in rural areas and proposed enlisting the state's Office of Public Health and the Tulane School of Public Health in this effort.

- In Virginia, leaders of the Turning Point initiative, convinced that local citizens should be consulted about what public health needs they considered most important, planned to establish teams to hold regional forums.

- In Nebraska, where less than a quarter of the state's counties provided any measure of public health service, the over-riding challenge was to develop a plan that would expand public health services throughout the state.

- In New Hampshire, which also suffered from a lack of a functioning public health system at the local level and where most of the state's 234 cities and towns employed health officers whose only qualification for the job was that they be residents of the state, the Turning Point initiative proposed forming coalitions of towns to pool resources, thereby expanding public health services.

—w— The National Excellence Collaboratives

In October 1999, The Robert Wood Johnson Foundation authorized an additional $15 million to carry out the implementation phase of the Turning Point initiative and, within it, to develop a number of National Excellence Collaboratives. Bobbie Berkowitz, the national program director, and Susan Hassmiller, a senior program officer at The Robert Wood Johnson Foundation who has overseen the program since 1997, had identified certain recurrent issues that cut across state lines and required special attention. Among them were the need for (1) acquiring better information and technology systems, (2) updating public health laws, (3) improving the performance management of local public health systems, (4) developing leadership, and (5) adopting commercial marketing techniques to persuade people to change unhealthy behaviors, such as cigarette smoking and drug abuse. As a result, The Robert Wood Johnson Foundation decided to create five National Excellence Collaboratives. Consisting of representatives from each state partnership and community partners, the collaboratives were charged with analyzing the five issues in greater detail and developing models that would provide solutions.

The states applying for implementation phase grants were given the opportunity of participating in up to two of the National Excellence Collaboratives. They could also apply to be the lead state for a particular collaborative, in which case they were required to show considerable expertise in the topic. States that were selected as participants in a National Excellence Collaborative received an additional grant of $150,000, and states designated as leaders of a collaborative received a supplementary $150,000.

The collaboratives met four times a year over the next four years.

- The Information Technology Collaborative developed an on-line Public Health Information Technology Catalogue to help community health agencies make decisions about which data systems could best meet their information needs.
- The Leadership Development Collaborative produced a core curriculum for leadership training and a set of leadership self-assessment tools.

■ The Performance Management Collaborative, after testing a four-part model in two states, developed a performance management tool kit.

■ The Social Marketing Collaborative designed a social marketing CD ROM based on work done by the Centers for Disease Control and Prevention. It was tested in two programs—one to promote the adoption of public health careers in Minnesota and the other to promote effective diabetes management in Virginia.

■ The Public Health Statute Modernization Collaborative contracted with the Center for Law and the Public's Health at Georgetown and Johns Hopkins Universities, which drafted the Turning Point Model State Public Health Act.[6] As of January 28, 2004, twenty-two states had introduced legislative bills or resolutions containing some of the provisions found in the model law, and sixteen of these bills had passed. However, because of provisions allowing for substantial increases in governmental powers to detect and contain bioterrorism threats or naturally occurring disease outbreaks, the model law has come under attack by a number of health professionals and civil liberties groups.[7]

—ᴡᴡ— The Implementation Phase

In March 2000, The Robert Wood Johnson Foundation awarded four-year implementation grants totaling $500,000 to each of the thirteen states—all but New Mexico—that had received planning grants and submitted public health improvement plans. (The seven states that had been awarded planning grants in the second wave of funding in 1999 received implementation grants in 2001.) Conversations with leaders of various Turning Point partnerships and visits to a number of states in the autumn of 2003 revealed the range of approaches that the partnerships had adopted to improve public health in their states.

Nebraska

In the first year of the implementation phase, only twenty-two of the state's ninety-three counties had local health departments. However, two community partnerships that were funded by the Kellogg Foundation—the North Central Community Care Partnership, a coalition of nine counties in the north central section of the state, and Buffalo County Community Health Partners, in the central region—implemented plans to address public health problems such as unhealthy aging, teen pregnancy, violence, obesity, poor water quality, and inadequate housing. Given the success of these efforts, the Nebraska Turning Point Project funded four new community-based partnerships in January 2001. Each of them received $15,000 from the Nebraska Turning Point Partnership, $15,000 in state matching funds, and a $10,000 local match.

The momentum generated by the Turning Point initiative helped to stimulate new public health legislation. In May 2001, the Nebraska legislature passed a law that appropriated $11.4 million from the state's Tobacco Settlement Fund to establish public health departments across the state over a two-year period. In addition, the law provided $5.6 million over a two-year period to address minority health needs, such as those reflected in disparate rates of infant mortality, cardiovascular disease, and diabetes.[8] By the summer of 2003, a wholesale transformation of Nebraska's public health infrastructure had occurred through the establishment of sixteen new multicounty public health departments that now provide public health services in all of the state's ninety-four counties.

David Palm, who is the administrator and coordinator of the Turning Point Initiative in the Nebraska Health and Human Services System, is proud of the achievements of Nebraska Turning Point, but aware that much remains to be done. "For the past two years, we've been holding statewide workshops to train the members of our newly established county departments of health in how to assess public health needs, develop policy, and diagnose problems," he said not long ago.

> Like other states, we're using bioterrorism money—in our case, $3 million of the $9 million we received in 2003 from the Center for Disease Control and Prevention's Emergency Preparedness Fund—to strengthen our public health

infrastructure. For example, we have used bioterrorism funds to buy fax machines, computers, and cell phones for our multicounty health departments so that their members can communicate effectively with one another in the event of attack. Among our unsolved problems are drinking-water contamination caused by pesticide pollution of wells and rivers, as well as by waste products from hog-confinement lots. Unfortunately, Nebraska's state and local health departments do not have sufficient regulatory power to deal adequately with this situation.

New Hampshire

Like Nebraska, New Hampshire has long been saddled with a fragmented and inadequate local public health system. Indeed, the first report deploring the lack of public health capacity in the state was issued back in 1883. In 1995, the state Department of Health and Human Services arranged for the creation of The Community Health Institute, a nonprofit organization that was originally charged with improving access to primary health care. Two years later, the Community Health Institute and the New Hampshire Public Health Association responded to The Robert Wood Johnson Foundation's call for proposals to join the Turning Point initiative. With the Institute acting as the Foundation's primary grantee, the two organizations took the lead in developing a public health improvement plan that gave priority to developing local public health coalitions.

By 1999, a new commissioner of the New Hampshire Department of Health and Human Services had been appointed, and Dr. William Kassler, formerly the director of a health services and evaluation program at the CDC, had been named state medical director. "When I arrived in New Hampshire at the end of 1998, I became involved in a battle taking place in two cities over whether a drinking-water fluoridation initiative should be placed on the ballot," Kassler said not long ago. "One city had a strong health department; the other had a weak one. In the city with the strong department, the initiative got on the ballot and was eventually approved. In the city with the weak department, the initiative failed to get on the ballot. It was an object lesson I haven't forgotten."

From the beginning, Kassler has proven to be a powerful supporter of the New Hampshire Turning Point initiative, whose leaders launched the program by competitively selecting four public health coalitions covering thirty-seven New Hampshire towns to receive funding and technical support. Most of these towns had large numbers of residents without health insurance, without adequate transportation to health care facilities, with poor dental care, and with annual family incomes that were well below the state average. One of the four public health coalitions was the North Country Health Consortium—a collection of thirty-five rural northern New Hampshire towns—whose members completed a health needs assessment and a public health improvement plan, and then used a grant from the New Hampshire Turning Point Initiative and the state to set up a mobile dental laboratory and develop a tobacco prevention program. The consortium also established the Northern New Hampshire Area Health Education Center, which trains health professionals in how to deal with diabetes, identify victims of domestic violence, screen for breast cancer, improve communication with patients, and care for terminally ill patients and those with dementia.

Kassler persuaded his former colleagues at the Centers for Disease Control and Prevention that CDC Health Alert Network funds could best be employed to strengthen local public health departments, and these funds were used to strengthen other health coalitions in the state. He also persuaded the state Department of Health and Human Services to create local initiatives with several million dollars of the $10 million in bioterrorism and emergency preparedness funds the state received from the CDC. At the same time, under the leadership of Jonathan Stewart, director of The Community Health Institute, Turning Point funds were used to provide training and technical assistance to the regional coalitions. At the end of 2003, the Turning Point coalitions had become the New Hampshire Public Health Network, and the collaboratives were serving eighty-seven communities and more than 60 percent of the state's residents. Future plans call for the expansion of the Public Health Network until all of the state's 234 towns and their residents are covered.

New York State

Unlike Nebraska and New Hampshire, New York State has had a long-established public health system that includes health departments in fifty-eight of its sixty-two counties (a single health department covers all five counties [boroughs] of New York City), and health commissioners who are physicians in the twelve largest counties—those with more than 250,000 residents. In 1998, the state received a Turning Point planning grant from The Robert Wood Johnson Foundation, and funding from the Kellogg Foundation for local public health partnerships in the five boroughs of New York City, in Chautauqua county, and in the Capital District counties of Albany, Rensselaer, and Schenectady. Over the next two years, priorities and strategies for strengthening the public health system were developed by members of the New York State Department of Health, the New York State Community Health Partnership (the name given to the state's Turning Point initiative), and the three local partnerships. At the conclusion of the planning phase, a steering committee selected training to improve the skills of the members of the public health workforce and of community health coalitions as the primary goal of New York's Turning Point initiative. In April 2000, New York State was awarded a four-year $950,000 Turning Point implementation grant to provide workforce training, participate in and lead the Social Marketing National Excellence Collaborative, and participate in the Collaborative on Performance Management.

Initially, New York State thought that an independent community health institute would be the most suitable way to provide public health training and education. During the second year of the implementation phase, however, it was decided that this training and education could best be provided by working within the New York State Department of Health system in collaboration with a number of academic and professional organizations, including the State University of New York, or SUNY, Albany School of Public Health, the New York and New Jersey Public Health Training Center, the New York State Nurses Association, and the New York State Association of County Health Officials. These institutions offer a wide-ranging public health curriculum that includes orientations for county health commissioners and public health directors, basic courses in public health, programs in environmental health, and training for public health nurses in community health assessment. The New York State Department of Health allocates $650,000 to SUNY Albany for much of this training.

According to Sylvia Pirani, who is director of the New York State Community Health Partnership, as well as of the New York State Health Department's Office of Local Health Services, one of the most successful of the training initiatives has been the Third Thursday Breakfast Broadcasts, known as T2B2, which were begun in 1999. "There are more than 12,000 public health workers in the New York State Department of Health and in the fifty-eight health departments in the state," Pirani said. "Many of these practitioners are eager to stay abreast of current public health issues, such as West Nile virus, Lyme disease, smallpox, SARS, lead poisoning, emergency preparedness, and biological threats such as anthrax, but have little time or resources for travel to meetings and workshops. The Third Thursday one-hour broadcasts have addressed the problem with a format that features a professional moderator interviewing a public health expert on a specific subject, and includes time for telephoned or faxed questions during the final ten minutes of the program. Satellite technology has made it possible to distribute the program nationally, and, thanks to financial support provided by the New York State Department of Health, the broadcasts now reach a live audience of up to 300 public health practitioners each month."

Virginia

The Commonwealth of Virginia established a board of health in 1872, and is one of a dozen or so states that operate a state-supervised public health system at the local level. The Virginia Department of Health serves the commonwealth through a central office in Richmond and thirty-five health districts made up of 119 city and county health departments throughout the state. Some of the health districts are made up of one city, such as Richmond, while other districts, such as the Three Rivers Health District, may contain up to ten counties. Each of them is directed by a full-time physician.

Virginia has chosen to reorganize its public health system by emphasizing collaboration between the public and private sectors. For example, the Virginia Department of Health elected to submit a joint proposal for Turning Point funding with the Virginia Hospital Research & Education

Foundation, a subsidiary of the Virginia Hospital & Healthcare Association, which is a statewide trade association that enjoys considerable clout with members of the Virginia state legislature. As further evidence of Virginia's bent toward a public/private partnership, the Department of Health asked the Hospital Research & Education Foundation to serve as the fiscal agent for Turning Point funds.[9]

During the Virginia Turning Point planning phase, the members of a steering committee identified several goals and methods for improving the commonwealth's public health system. Among them were conducting a community health needs assessment, developing public awareness about health issues, assessing the economics of disease prevention programs, emphasizing the use of information-based health decisions, and enhancing the skills of the public health workforce. To reach these goals, Virginia Turning Point officials recommended the formation of a new partnership that would also serve as a vehicle for building bridges with the business sector. In March 2000, urged on by the efforts of the Virginia Hospital & Healthcare Association, the Virginia Legislature authorized the creation of the Virginia Center for Healthy Communities, which was established as a nonprofit 501(c)(3) entity. The center's board of trustees was made up of members from public and private entities, whose mission included forging "a stronger link between the interests of the business and health sectors," on the assumption that the two have "common goals of effective interventions that are cost effective."[10]

Whether the public/private partnership that characterizes the Virginia Center for Healthy Communities is improving the public health of the Commonwealth is not yet known, because, as with Turning Point initiatives in other states, it is too early to measure outcomes. According to Jeffrey Wilson, who is the coordinator of Turning Point and Strategic Planning for the Virginia Department of Health, an early success has been the *Virginia Atlas of Community Health*. The *Atlas* is a Web-based interactive map that contains county and ZIP-code-level data for 114 population, economic, and health indicators in Virginia. It enables planners and health officials to identify health needs in specific neighborhoods. "This kind of mapping allows decision makers to focus their efforts on localities where the health needs are most acute," Wilson says. "For example, we can use data from the *Atlas* to approach asthma victims and train them how to manage their asthma attacks without using hospital emergency rooms. Data from the *Atlas* can also help us determine where problems like diabetes are most acute, and that information can help us target resources to the areas of greatest need."

South Carolina

South Carolina ranks as one of the nation's five worst states in terms of health indicators, including very high rates of mortality from stroke and heart disease and of HIV/AIDS. Moreover, persistent disparities exist between African Americans and whites living in the state. Not surprising, members of the South Carolina Department of Health and Environmental Control were disappointed when The Robert Wood Johnson and Kellogg Foundations turned down its initial application for a Turning Point planning phase grant. However, the state was able to provide $150,000 for strategic planning to improve South Carolina's public health system, in the event that the application for Turning Point funding was rejected, which meant that the planning phase was able to proceed on its own. Thanks largely to this extracurricular effort, which was spearheaded by Lisa Waddell, deputy commissioner for health services, and Jerry Dell Gimarc, senior planner in the health department's planning office, The Robert Wood Johnson and the Kellogg Foundations approved South Carolina's second application for Turning Point funding in June of 1999.

A department of health official for twenty-four years, Dell Gimarc has directed the state's Turning Point initiative since the beginning. When she retired from the health department in 2000, she moved to the University of South Carolina Center for Health Services and Policy Research, which the department had designated as the fiscal agent for Turning Point. "South Carolina's public health system is strong and well integrated, with health departments in each of the state's forty-six counties that are affiliated with one of twelve multicounty health districts," she said recently. "What we wanted to accomplish with Turning Point was to strengthen local health departments." "Our chief goals have been to improve the competency of our workforce and to reach out to our communities and engage their support," added deputy commissioner Waddell. "Thanks largely to health department funds, we've sent forty-six health professionals to train at the University of North Carolina Public Health Leadership Institute. With funding from the Centers for Disease Control and Prevention, we've enrolled 249 health officers in an executive education course at the University's Management Academy for Public Health." During the planning stage, which took place from 1999 to 2001, funds from The Robert Wood Johnson Foundation were used to support pilot projects in Anderson County in the northwest part of the state, Horry County in the east, and Hampton County in the south. South Carolina's Turning Point is currently using its implementation grant funds to support partnerships in six additional counties.

—⟋⟍— Controversies and Issues

As might be expected, an undertaking of the magnitude and complexity of Turning Point did not occur without engendering some controversy and raising fundamental issues. The main issues concern the conceptual bases of the program, the way it was implemented, and, in a broader public health context, the use of bioterrorism funds for public health purposes.

The Conceptual Bases of the Turning Point Initiative

A number of academics have questioned the basic premises of Turning Point. They have wondered whether, in endeavoring to transform public health, the program was oversold; whether collaboration would bring about improvements in the public's health; and whether partnership of government with the private sector was desirable or realistic. Many of these questions were raised in the January 2002 issue of the *Journal of Public Health Management and Practice,* which was devoted to exploring the Turning Point Initiative.

In that issue of the *Journal,* Rebecca Socolar, clinical associate professor of pediatrics and social medicine at the University of North Carolina School of Medicine at Chapel Hill, reviewed three articles written by Turning Point officials and found that the authors had failed to make clear whether collaboration—the quintessential mantra of Turning Point—was a goal in and of itself or a tool to use toward achieving improvement in public health. "Part of the problem is that until a group has defined its goals explicitly and clearly, the desired outcome may be so nebulous that it is unclear what tools may be useful in reaching those goals," Socolar wrote. "Goals such as 'creating a new approach to community health' or 'improving health' are so vague that it is unclear what exactly the goals are and unclear what processes are best to achieve these goals." She concluded by observing that "there still needs to be better evidence about outcomes related to collaboration."[11]

Stephen Linder, associate professor of management and policy sciences at the School of Public Health of the University of Texas, in Houston, questioned the basic premise of public-private collaboration and the borrowing of private sector practices for public health purposes. Such borrowing, he wrote, favored "private over public provision of services and market virtues over government responsibilities," and he predicted that after privatization in businesslike partnerships, "public health would be 'branded' like laundry soap and promoted to communities of customers." Moreover, he said that the articles he had reviewed echoed the promotional tone of materials disseminated by The Robert Wood Johnson and Kellogg foundations, and were written in a bewildering and self-congratulatory language he referred to as 'TurningPointSpeak.'"[12]

Peter Jacobson, associate professor in the Health Management and Policy Department at the University of Michigan School of Public Health, in Ann Arbor, questioned the strategy of public-private collaboration and the motives of the private sector for participating in public health partnerships. "Will they co-opt public resources without providing adequate services, leaving a void?" he asked. "Or will they simply overwhelm the public sector, only to abandon the field when it becomes inopportune? After the public sector is dismantled, it will be very difficult to put back together."[13]

Another conceptual issue is whether the public health infrastructure is so weak that, despite the best efforts of the Turning Point initiative, it will remain subject to political and commercial pressures and unable to carry out significant aspects of its mandate, such as addressing environmental health problems in a timely fashion. In some cases, this is because health departments are separate entities from departments of the environment. In other cases, political or commercial interests have managed to thwart health department officials from addressing environmental health issues. The aftermath of September 11th offers a dramatic illustration. A week after the terrorist attacks on the World Trade Center, the White House Council on Environmental Quality downplayed the tremendous environmental health problems in lower Manhattan, and the Environmental Protection Agency declared that the air in lower Manhattan was safe to breathe. The public health leadership in New York City did not protest, despite the high levels of asbestos and other toxins in the air and on the ground that threatened the health of workers and residents and whose harmful effects have since been demonstrated in a number of reports.[14]

Implementation

As happens with many programs—especially those relying on the formation and work of coalitions—implementation was not rapid or smooth. The Robert Wood Johnson Foundation's Susan Hassmiller has noted, "The process has been slow and tedious. It's hard to break down public health barriers. Neither side—public health on the one side and others, such as business, on the other—has much incentive to work with the other. Also it is cumbersome for agencies within state government to work in a collaborative fashion." In the case of Turning Point, implementation was made even more difficult by the divergent cultures of the two foundations that had conceived of the initiative.

The cultural differences between Kellogg and Robert Wood Johnson became apparent almost from the start. "Kellogg is a grassroots kind of organization, really interested in the community," Bobbie Berkowitz has said. "Robert Wood Johnson is more large-scale, systems-oriented, and interested in having a major impact nationally." Marilyn Aguirre-Molina, who left The Robert Wood Johnson Foundation to become a professor of public health at Columbia University's Mailman School of Public Health, explained that "Kellogg initially wanted to give local health departments very wide latitude about what they could do under Turning Point," whereas "Robert Wood Johnson had a tendency to let the health departments know what results it expected them to achieve."[15]

Because of such cultural differences, teams from the two foundations charged with selecting state and community sites had a difficult time coming to agreement. Moreover, when agreement was reached, the initial fourteen state and forty-one community grantees were placed on different timetables. For example, The Robert Wood Johnson Foundation authorized only two years of funding for the planning phase, while agreeing to consider additional funds for more sites and for an implementation phase at a later time, whereas the Kellogg Foundation authorized three years of funding up front for both planning and implementation. Tension between the two foundations was further exacerbated in October 1998 when, without alerting The Robert Wood Johnson Foundation, NACCHO, the national program office for the Kellogg Foundation's part of Turning Point, sent a letter to the forty-one Kellogg Foundation grantees stating that because of a stock market decline that reduced Kellogg's endowment, their activities might have to be curtailed.

To salvage a deteriorating situation, Susan Hassmiller suggested holding a retreat for key staff members from both institutions and their respective national program offices. The participants in the meeting, which took place in Chicago in August 1999, agreed upon a plan of regular communications that alleviated many of the interfoundation problems. However, certain inherent weaknesses in Turning Point remained difficult to overcome. Gloria Smith of the Kellogg Foundation has pointed out that "it would have been far better for both foundations to have been on the same timetable from the start and to plan the program around a common framework."[16] Vincent Lafronza, Turning Point program director at NACCHO, believes that the financing of the initiative was flawed from the beginning. "States and communities should have been financed jointly and allowed to agree together on how to use the money," he says. "Instead, when it came to funding the implementation grants, Kellogg and Robert Wood Johnson acted independently of each other in selecting the communities they would finance. This, of course, was antithetical to the basic premise of Turning Point, which was to encourage collaboration."

The Use of Bioterrorism Funds

Since the terrorist attacks of September 11, 2001, nearly $1 billion in federal grants has been made available to state and local health departments to enhance public health preparedness to handle a range of potential public health emergencies.[17] Two schools of thought have emerged as to whether this huge influx of federal money focused on bioterrorism has been beneficial or harmful to the overall goals of Turning Point. Some experts, such as Jeffrey Koplan, vice president for academic health affairs at the Woodruff Health Sciences Center at Emory University and former head of the CDC, argue that strategies developed in response to bioterrorism threats expand the ability of state public health departments to fulfill their broader mission to protect against a full range of risks to the public's health. "The tools we develop in response to bioterrorism threats are 'dual use' tools," he wrote. "Not only will they ensure that we are prepared for man-made threats, but they also ensure that we will be able to recognize and control the naturally emerging infectious diseases and the hazardous materials incidences of the late 20th century."[18]

Others believe that the overriding focus on bioterrorism siphons money and public health personnel away from arguably greater threats and from broad community partnerships capable of addressing a wide variety of public health issues. Victor Sidel and Barry Levy, both past presidents of the American Public Health Association, assert that extraordinary political and economic pressures have subverted sound public health principles in favor of addressing the threat of bioterrorism, and that urgent problems are being neglected.[19]

Clearly, the challenge posed by the current national preoccupation with bioterrorisim is something that state health departments will have to deal with if they are to carry out their essential mission of preventing and controlling disease. The challenge affects, and is affected by, Turning Point. As Betty Bekemeier, deputy director of the Turning Point National Program Office, and Jan Dahl, a senior consultant to Turning Point, noted, "the strong relationship between bioterrorism preparedness planning and the broader concepts of public health system development include issues such as local capacity building, information technology infrastructures, and workforce development"—the very basics of the Turning Point program.[20]

—⁓— Conclusions

Turning Point is an ambitious initiative with the admirable if somewhat amorphous goal of improving the public health systems of states, counties, and communities through the development of collaborative partnerships between public health departments, other state and local health agencies, schools of public health, the business community, health maintenance organizations, environmental coalitions, and faith-based groups. The premise behind Turning Point holds promise, not least of all because of the enthusiasm and the dedication of the initiative's participants across the nation—an enthusiasm and dedication that can be found from those working in the north woods of New Hampshire to those toiling in isolated and impoverished counties of South Carolina.

On December 16 and 17, 2003, eighty-five public health leaders—among them representatives of The Robert Wood Johnson Foundation, the Turning Point national program offices, state Turning Point directors, national public health organizations, and business executives—met at the Foundation's headquarters, in Princeton, New Jersey, to discuss what had been learned and accomplished during the six-year initiative.

At this meeting, the program's evaluators, Todd Rogers and Dianne Barker of the Public Health Institute, summarized the major themes they observed in the course of their qualitative evaluation of the Turning Point initiative. They pointed out that new structures had expanded the ability of a number of Turning Point states to respond to public health issues, among them:

- The creation of offices dedicated to public health improvement in state health departments in Montana, Nebraska, Oklahoma, and Wisconsin
- The establishment of public health institutes outside of state health departments in Illinois, Louisiana, Missouri, and Virginia

■ The expansion of local public health systems through government structures in Nebraska and Nevada and through partnerships in Minnesota, New Hampshire, and Oklahoma

Rogers and Barker also cited the work done by some of the National Excellence Collaborations, and described efforts by several states to institute enhanced leadership programs and to expand training opportunities in order to provide a more competent public health workforce.

The meeting's participants agreed that Turning Point had transformed the way people think about public health in terms of partnership, culture change, and the need to improve public health systems. They emphasized the importance of partnerships in lessening the impact of state budget cuts, and of communication as a way of overcoming the generally poor understanding of public health by members of the general population. The Robert Wood Johnson Foundation's Hassmiller suggested that one of the initiative's legacies would be the creation of public institutes in many states. "These nonprofit institutes," she said, "work with state and local government health departments to get work done in a more expeditious fashion than government can do alone."

Turning Point has already made significant progress by helping to enlarge the scope of public health systems, especially in states such as Nebraska and New Hampshire, where dozens of multitown and multicounty partnerships have been formed to provide public health services to populations that were previously deprived of them; by facilitating the education and training of public health professionals through such methods as New York State's monthly radio broadcasts; and by compiling data on community health status as exemplified by the *Virginia Atlas of Community Health*.

In spite of its achievements, the jury is still out on Turning Point, for a number of reasons. First, after only four years of implementation funding, it is too early to know whether the progress made so far in states and communities can be sustained in the face of huge budget cuts that are taking place at all levels of government across the nation. Second, it is questionable whether public health coalitions and better trained public health officials will be any better equipped than their predecessors to stand up to the powerful political and commercial interests opposing their efforts. Third, there is as yet no hard evidence to support the premise that the public-private-nongovernmental collaboration that lies at the heart of the Turning Point vision will result in improving the health of the public.

Finally, the contributions of Turning Point's partnerships at the state and community level must be seen in the context of a public health system that the Institute of Medicine described in 1988 as being in "disarray"[21] and, in 2003, found to be characterized by "vulnerable and outdated health information systems and technologies, an insufficient and inadequately trained public health workforce, antiquated laboratory capacity, a lack of real-time surveillance and epidemiological systems, ineffective and fragmented communications networks, incomplete domestic preparedness and emergency response capabilities, and communities without access to essential public health services."[22] While Turning Point has produced valuable insights and changes in a number of states and communities, the challenge of transforming the public health system is an enormous one. Meeting it will require not only the efforts of foundations like Robert Wood Johnson and Kellogg but also a transformation of the public's awareness of the importance of public health to the nation.

Notes

1. Institute of Medicine. *The Future of Public Health.* Washington, D.C.: National Academy Press, 1988, p. 19.
2. Ibid., p. 19.
3. Ibid, pp. 139–155.
4. Hassmiller, S. "Turning Point: The Robert Wood Johnson Foundation's Effort to Revitalize Public Health at the State Level." *Journal of Public Health Management and Practice,* 2002, 8(1), 4.
5. The first director of the program was Gilbert Omenn. Berkowitz became program director when Omenn left in 1997.
6. The Model Act was drafted in October 2001 in collaboration with the National Governors Association, the National Conference of State Legislatures, the National Association of Attorneys General, the Association of State and Territorial Health Officials, and the National Association of County and City Health Officials.

Transformations in Public Health, Spring 2002, *4*(1), 1. Turning Point National Program Office, University of Washington, Seattle.

7. Sidel, V. W., and Levy, B. S. "Policy Corner." *Transformations in Public Health,* Winter, 2003, *4*(4), 10. Turning Point National Program Office, University of Washington, Seattle.

8. Palm, D. "Building a Sustainable Public Infrastructure in Nebraska." *Transformations in Public Health,* Autumn 2001, *3*(4), 7–8.

9. Lake, J. L., and Peterson, E. A. "An Alternative Structure for Improving the Public's Health." *Journal of Public Health Management and Practice,* 2002, *8*(1), 77.

10. Ibid., pp. 80–81.

11. Socolar, R. "Collaboration: The End or the Means?" *Journal of Public Health Management and Practice,* 2002, *8,* 34.

12. Linder, S. H. "On the Politics of Policy Development." *Journal of Public Health Management and Practice,* 2002, *8,* 62–63

13. Jacobson, P. D. "Form Versus Function in Public Health." *Journal of Public Health Management and Practice,* 2002, *8,* 92–93.

14. DePalma, A. "Many Who Served on 9/11 Are Still Pressing the Fight for Workers' Compensation." *New York Times,* May 13, 2004, A24; Kennedy, R. F., Jr. "The Junk Science of George W. Bush." *The Nation,* March 8, 2004; Pope, C. "Whitewash at Ground Zero: How the White House Covered Up Post-September 11 Hazards." *Sierra Magazine,* January/February 2004.

15. Isaacs, S. L., and Rodgers, J. H. "Partnership Among National Foundations." *To Improve Health and Health Care, 2001: The Robert Wood Johnson Foundation Anthology.* San Francisco: Jossey-Bass, 2001, p. 232.

16. Isaacs, S. L., and Rodgers, J. H. "Partnership Among National Foundations." *To Improve Health and Health Care, 2001: The Robert Wood Johnson Foundation Anthology.* San Francisco: Jossey-Bass, 2001, p. 233.

17. Bekemeier, B., and Dahl, J. "Turning Point Sets the Stage for Emergency Preparedness Planning." *Journal of Health Management and Practice,* 2003, *9,* 377–383.

18. Koplan, J. "Policy Corner." *Transformations in Public Health,* Winter 2003, *4*(4), 10. Turning Point National Program Office, University of Washington, Seattle.

19. Sidel, V. W., and Levy, B. S. "Policy Corner." *Transformations in Public Health,* Winter 2003, *4*(4), 10. Turning Point National Program Office, University of Washington, Seattle.

20. Bekemeier, B., and Dahl, J. "Turning Point Sets the Stage for Emergency Preparedness Planning." *Journal of Public Health Management Practice,* 2003, *9,* 377–383.

21. Institute of Medicine. *The Future of Public Health.* Washington, D.C.: National Academy Press, 1988.

22. Ibid., page 3.

A Closer Look

CHAPTER

6

The Chicago Project
for Violence Prevention

Digby Diehl

Editors' Introduction

Every year, *The Robert Wood Johnson Foundation Anthology* contains a chapter that looks at one of the smaller investments made by the Foundation. This close look at a community project is meant to provide a balance to the attention generally given to the Foundation's large, multisite national initiatives, and to put a human face on its programs. Although 65 percent of the Foundation's approximately $400 million annual payout goes to these national initiatives, the Foundation makes between 240 and 427 grants annually to projects outside of these large national initiatives. Many of the grants are based on unsolicited ideas developed and advanced by creative people interested in addressing a health-related problem. In addition, the Foundation supports the Local Initiative Funding Partners Program, which, in collaboration with other, primarily local, foundations, makes grants to support community-based organizations and community-generated ideas.

The Chicago Project for Violence Prevention is one of the projects funded by the Local Initiative Funding Partners Program—in this case, in partnership with the Chicago-based John D. and Catherine T. MacArthur Foundation and the Chicago Community Trust. The brainchild of the physician-epidemiologist Gary Slutkin, who dedicated himself to doing something about the striking number of homicides involving Chicago children, the project strives to reduce violence in high-crime, gang-ridden neighborhoods. The project is unusual in two respects. First, it evolved from Slutkin's experience in East Africa, and represents one of those occasions when the developed world learns from the developing world. Second, violence prevention is not one of The Robert Wood Johnson Foundation's priorities. However, the project turned out to be such an interesting one that it was awarded an almost unprecedented second grant from the Local Initiative Funding Partners Program.

Digby Diehl, the author of this chapter, is a frequent contributor to *The Robert Wood Johnson Foundation Anthology* series. Diehl did his research on the chapter by spending time with the principal actors in the project and witnessing their work on the streets of Chicago.

—ɯ— **M**any Americans were astonished to learn in the movie *Bowling for Columbine* that more than 11,000 people are killed by guns in the United States each year, and another 16,000 people use a gun to commit suicide.[1] Compared with thirty-six other industrialized nations, the United States is the world leader in gun death by a wide margin. In Japan, for example, a citizen is 208 times less likely to be killed by a gun than in the United States.[2] In its first ever *World Report on Violence and Health,* the World Health Organization reported in 2002 that more than 1.6 million people worldwide are killed by violence every year.[3] Violence is one of the leading causes of death among people aged fifteen to forty-four, and it accounts for 14 percent of deaths among males and 7 percent of deaths among females. Each day around the globe, more than 1,400 people are killed in acts of homicide—almost one person every minute.[4]

In Illinois, the number of people killed by guns jumped 14 percent, from 1,130 in 2000 to 1,289 in 2001.[5] According to the Chicago Police Department, the city had 598 homicides in 2003, down 8 percent from 2002.[6] Unfortunately, this still made Chicago's murder rate approximately four times the national rate. The city has both the highest murder rate of the nine largest cities in the United States and the highest number of homicides. Of the 598 homicides in Chicago in 2003, 484, or 81 percent, were committed with a gun.[7]

—ɯ— "Children Shooting Other Children with Guns"

These grim statistics are the backdrop for the creation of the Chicago Project for Violence Prevention, which was founded by physician Gary Slutkin in 1995. A Chicago native, Slutkin returned to his hometown after two decades of moving around the world as an epidemiologist. As chief of interventions and prevention for the World Health Organization, he had battled tuberculosis in San Francisco and Somalia, AIDS in Uganda, and other infectious diseases internationally. By 1994, Slutkin was ready to come home. "I had been traveling from country to country for years, and I was in my forties," Slutkin recalls. "But what was I going to do? There are plenty of AIDS doctors in the United States. In fact, it didn't seem as though the U.S. had any problems at all: everybody has clean water piped into their homes; there is a lot of food; the land is good; the GNP is enormous. Then, gradually, people began to tell me about the situation of children shooting other children with guns."

On first returning to the United States in 1994, Slutkin spent six months in Washington, D.C., talking with government leaders about the growing problem of violence in our cities. After returning to Chicago, he questioned city officials, police administrators, university professors, priests and ministers, community leaders, gang members, and prisoners. He then repeated the process in several other cities. He was disturbed by how intractable the problem of violence in our inner cities seemed to be, and by how ineffective most of the efforts to cope with it had been. "I listened to hundreds of stories about ten-year-olds shooting twelve-year-olds, and about how incredibly unsafe American cities were becoming. I had heard nothing like that overseas—except for war zones," Slutkin says. "There were all kinds of programs and projects, but I didn't see a city that really had a strategy for reducing violent behavior—certainly not one that made any sense. I was touched by the stories I heard and puzzled by the problem. It seemed to me that this was a terrible trend that had to be reversed. Chicago, my hometown, was the national epicenter for violence, so I decided to begin here. I got support for my own salary and then an assistant and finally some staff. We just rolled up our sleeves and began."

Susan Scrimshaw, dean of the School of Public Health at the University of Illinois at Chicago, immediately saw the importance of Slutkin's determined focus. His colleagues at the department of epidemiology at the university were equally willing to support his new project, even though no one—including Slutkin—really knew what it would be or how it would function. Installed in offices at the School of Public Health, Slutkin began drawing upon his experiences with epidemics in Somalia, Uganda, and sub-Saharan Africa. Others have used words such as "epidemic" and "disease" as metaphors to explain problems of violence. Slutkin sees violence as literally a public health issue, a social disease that may respond to the same preventive practices that he has applied to epidemics in many parts of the world.

"If you trace our whole global history as human beings, all you see is failure in the realm of violence prevention," Slutkin observes. "Our whole history is one of wars. The last century was the most violent ever, and the last decade had the largest war since World War II, in which two and a half million people died in the Congo, as well as genocide in Bosnia, Kosovo, and Rwanda."

Slutkin finds that the twenty-first century has not begun well either, with terrorist attacks and war becoming more and more common. "Thus far, our response to violence has been more violence," he says. "That's why the idea of approaching the problem of violence as a health problem seems so revolutionary. The general public believes: one, there's nothing you can do about it; two, violent behavior is 'natural' to the perpetrators; and three, the appropriate response is to put them in prison or some other form of retaliation. I believe that this public perception is wrong on all counts."

"Kids who behave violently have learned this behavior," Slutkin says.

> They have learned it from their parents, from their peers, from the police, from their entertainment, from their communities. For them, violence is simply a cultural norm. We need to change that norm. Whatever you're talking about—smoking behavior, drunk-driving behavior, seat belt behavior, immunizing behavior, breast-feeding behavior, condom-using behavior—these are areas where societies have successfully changed norms that affect public health. Not every culture agrees that you should not have unprotected sex, or should not have ten or twelve children in each family, or should not be free to smoke in public places. On the other hand, almost everyone agrees that we should not have violence. This is an easier behavior to change. If you provide some alternatives, some modeling, some handholding, some safe retreat and face-saving, you can change people. It's only a behavioral norm.

—〰— A Place to Begin: Identifying Infrastructure

In the early years of the Chicago Project for Violence Prevention, Slutkin worked with a small team to build alliances with organizations already working in the most violent neighborhoods. "Public health people talk about building on existing infrastructures, and I really believe it," he says. "In African refugee camps, people would say, 'Oh, there's no infrastructure here.' Well, there is. You just can't see it until you start to ask questions. The mothers talk to one another, and the tribes talk to one another, and the ethnic groups talk with one another. In an inner city situation, you want to discover the different community infrastructures. You want to learn who's working with whom and who doesn't want to work with whom. You need to develop relationships so that people are not automatically against you."

Slutkin and his small staff decided to focus initially on the Austin neighborhood, a predominately African American area that led all Chicago communities in the number of homicides in the mid-1990s, according to the Chicago Police Department. "What we looked for was a community group that had some relationship to the residents, had a recognized leadership, and had a desire to do something for the community in the area of violence prevention," Slutkin says.

In many other countries, you will find a government ministry. In U.S. cities, the infrastructure is primarily police, fire, and schools. Fire isn't really relevant here. Schools arguably could work, but primarily in the daytime. And police wasn't where we wanted it to begin. We were working on the streets, often in the evening and at night. What we began to look for was a community group to serve as a project partner. The Austin community actually had four community groups that worked together. As it turned out, we worked primarily with one group, and they worked well with the other three. The Austin community formed a violence-prevention coalition with youth groups and other social service agencies and police and probation; this became the model we followed in other communities. In each of the neighborhoods where we are involved, we work with one community group and try to form a coalition that is as all-inclusive as possible. From the community's point of view, the infrastructure is that already established community group.

Beginning in 1995 and working with the Austin Violence Prevention Consortium, the Chicago Project for Violence Prevention began to address the problem on a block-by-block basis, stabilizing one block as a peaceful area before adding another. It enhanced community policing with people who were given the task of identifying areas in the neighborhood where violence repeatedly erupted, and provided an aggressive program of public education with leaflets, posters, and classroom speakers. It also provided job opportunities and opened the Austin High School for after-school programs.

In 1997, the Chicago Project offered a summary of its activities in the first two years. First, the group had recruited a core of technical experts in violence prevention. Many of the people in the office had academic backgrounds; but the outreach workers were chosen for their abilities to relate to people in the community and to identify with problems on the streets—because they had lived with them personally. Second, they reviewed successful community programs that could serve as models and developed a strategy to adapt those models in the target communities. Slutkin believed wholeheartedly in the public health strategy: the idea that violence is a learned behavior and that epidemics of violence can be controlled by changing community behavioral norms.

In 1997, as the program began to show promise in the Austin community, the Grand Boulevard and Logan Square neighborhoods were added, and funding was found for a full-time violence prevention program manager in each neighborhood. In the office, a rigorous set of evaluation tools—using Chicago Police Department records of shootings and survey data—was developed. At the same time, a steering committee was formed. Consisting of representatives from all levels of the city of Chicago, the steering committee served as a citywide mechanism to support the specific communities with assistance from many partners in the city government to stop violence. It also provided linkages with the police and probation services.

As the Chicago Project for Violence Prevention found greater financial and political support for its efforts, it worked on developing different plans tailored to each neighborhood. It also provided modest funding and fund-raising assistance to selected youth and domestic violence prevention programs.

—ww— The Local Initiative Funding Partners Grant Application

By 1998, the Chicago Project had attracted the support of the Department of Justice, The Chicago Community Trust, and The John D. and Catherine T. MacArthur Foundation. In December of that year, Slutkin applied to the Local Initiative Funding Partners Program of The Robert Wood Johnson Foundation. The grant application proposed to expand the program over a four-year period, to eventually include a total of seven Chicago communities. These seven neighborhoods were at that time responsible for almost 40 percent of all homicides citywide.[8] The application predicted a dramatic reduction of forty to a hundred fewer killings per year at the end of the four-year period. Developed by the Chicago Project Steering Committee and consisting of twenty city, county, state, and federal agencies, the core of this violence prevention program is an eight-point plan:

1. Strong community-wide coalitions and community work on norms.

2. A unified message to those at the highest risk that shooting is out.

3. Rapid and coordinated response to any violence, including prevention of retaliating.

4. Identification of most at-risk persons and ensuring alternatives and linkages.

5. Additional supervision of those most at risk (including those on probation) for gun use and involvement in violence.

6. Increased availability, safety, use, and supervision of after-school programs, other safe havens.

7. Increasing pressure on guns and gun movement at all steps.

8. Prosecutions for violence and communication of prosecutions and sentences.

The application to the Local Initiative Funding Partners Program provided a detailed description of the plan and how it would be implemented, monitored, and evaluated. "When the grant proposal first came in, it was an unusual application for a Local Initiative project, because it positioned shooting and street violence as a public health issue," recalls Pauline Seitz, the director of the program. "Our reviewers spent considerable time debating whether this really fit into the context of our Local Initiatives program. It came to us with strong local support. The MacArthur Foundation and The Chicago Community Trust offered persuasive arguments that the problems of community violence were a significant public health issue. The costs within the local medical systems to deal with treatment and follow-up were substantial, not to mention the mental health consequences. It moved forward with debate from concept paper to full proposal. Finally, we made the decision that we should visit Chicago to learn more about the program."

"There was a remarkable level of cooperation from all parts of the communities brought together by the Chicago Project for Violence Prevention," Seitz recalls.

> The steering committee brought support from the top echelons of the city together with grassroots community groups. Often in collaborations of this size and scope, you have very strong ground support for it and very strong conceptual support at the policy level, but it is hard to pull the middle in. But they were doing it.
>
> One of the most impressive points made to us during the site visit was that if you lived in a neighborhood where a street light had been shot out, you would know whom to call and would get almost immediate attention to the problem. To me, that was a realistic example of how well the project could work.

The most powerful aspect of the Local Initiative site visit was a trip into the devastated neighborhoods that Slutkin proposed to serve. "As we visited these communities, there was no question that they were infected with drug abuse and violence," Seitz says.

> These are unsafe, unhealthy communities where the norm is violence. These are places where no one feels safe. The framing of it as a public health issue—that

the violence is contagious, that it has become an epidemic—was appropriate. When you put outreach workers into the situation, they can change community attitudes. The outreach model has been effective not only in American health situations but also in international health. It has ameliorated deep community health problems. Dr. Slutkin made a strong case that this could work and that Chicago was an environment where it needed to be tried. We decided to fund the project.

—∿— Lessons from the Boston CeaseFire Program

In addition to the development of the overall Chicago Project for Violence Prevention, the project supported by the Local Initiative Funding Partners Program included an innovation called CeaseFire. Adapted from a successful Boston antiviolence program, it focused on an intensified multiagency outreach effort, which involved the city, the police, the clergy, and other social agencies working in cooperation with one another. The Chicago Project people learned from Boston's experience that when agencies and individuals overcame their own turf warfare, they could accomplish more. As James T. Jordan, who was director of planning for the Boston Police Department, put it, "The key is collaboration."

Boston's program was impressive. A Harvard study identified about 1,300 young people in sixty-one gangs. Although they made up less than 1 percent of their age group citywide, they were responsible for at least 60 percent of all youth homicides in the city. Moreover, the violence was disproportionately clustered in gang turf.[9] Unlike Chicago, where violence often appears to be drug-related, Boston's violence was more personal and retributive. The initial study, directed by the senior researcher David Kennedy at the John F. Kennedy School of Government at Harvard University, defined the problem and helped determine the course of its solution. "The main message, backed up with posters and handouts was . . . from now on, when you do violence we are going to crack down on you on every available legal front."[10]

Coordinated by the Boston Police Department, this project, dubbed Operation CeaseFire, concentrated on identifying high-risk gang members and intervening among them to alter their behavior. Aided by a coalition of fifty-four churches called the Boston Ten-Point Coalition, the department deployed street workers, most of whom were ex-offenders themselves. One minister, the Reverend Eugene Rivers, is a former gang member who knows the territory. He has been effective in attracting troubled youths to the programs at his church's recreation center.[11]

In Boston, Operation CeaseFire is the end result of a planned intervention that has a number of organizations at its center. As Blaine Harden of the *Washington Post* reported, "When, for example, Boston's Youth Violence Strike Force decides to smash a boomlet of juvenile violence, they order an 'Operation CeaseFire,' which begins with a neighborhood meeting."[12] The Strike Force informs parents of the impending crackdown, and follows up with weekly police check-ins with the street workers, teachers, and other neighborhood leaders. These proactive measures are simultaneously accompanied by other initiatives—including heavy sentences for gun possession, intensive "no-violence" messages, and plenty of counseling coming from the clergy.

Slutkin saw how the Boston group drew together organizations to form a "community octopus" that embraced troubled and violent teenagers who, perhaps for the first time, heard the message that someone cares. "We added two components to the Boston plan," Slutkin says. "First, we designed a massive public education effort, a way of messaging to the community. It mobilizes people and gives them information for action, instead of feeling trapped. Second, the most important component of our project that is different from Boston's program is the strong emphasis on community involvement and community awareness. We work hard to make sure that people in the neighborhoods talk to one another. We added that to the efforts of police, clergy, and outreach workers."

The Chicago Project for Violence Prevention has also created a communications network, whereby the highest ranks of city government hear about street-level problems through regular project steering committee meetings. Chicago Mayor Richard Daley and Francis Cardinal George, the Archbishop of Chicago, are cochairs of the Chicago Project, and Slutkin notes that their involvement is not simply ceremonial: "We have regular contact with the mayor's office, and Cardinal George has taken the leadership of the Covenant for Peace in Action. Cardinal George personally mediated a solution to a gang warfare situation that undoubtedly saved lives." The Covenant for Peace in Action, signed by 122 Chicago clergy, commits its signatories to active participation in violence prevention measures, including urging congregations to respond to shootings, leading night marches, offering safe havens to victims, and mediating between violent groups.[13]

—⟋⟋⟍— Inside the Chicago Project for Violence Prevention Offices

At the nerve center of the Chicago Project for Violence Prevention, in offices on the tenth floor of the University of Illinois School of Public Health, a violence management team under the direction of Slutkin monitors shootings throughout Chicago on a twenty-four-hour basis. It alerts community action groups, coordinates crisis intervention, and supports seventy outreach workers in the field. The team shares the latest data in regular meetings, where so-called Rapid Response strategies are put into action. When a shooting is reported in one of the Chicago Project neighborhoods, churches, schools, and community organizations are asked to gather at the scene to express their disapproval publicly. The shooter receives the message from the community that his violent behavior is unacceptable. Perhaps equally important, large crowds of people, often staying around until late at night, are bad for drug sales. "Between twenty-four and seventy-two hours after a shooting," says Frank Perez, the project's outreach coordinator, "we inundate that spot with our "no shooting" materials, with our outreach workers, with church members, with clergy, and we walk." The ceremonies may involve prayer, setting up urban monuments, or holding rallies to drum up support for no violence.

Sending messages to the community is just as important as receiving messages from the community. "I have to tell people in a hundred different ways, over and over, to stop killing each other," says Stephanie Shapiro, public education coordinator for the project. The messages on her posters are strong and to the point:

- Stop. Killing. People.

- Don't Let 6 × 9 [the size of a prison cell] or 6 Feet Under Be Your Only Choices.

- What if you could take back the split second you pulled the trigger?

- Four to fifteen years for just shooting a gun. Is it really worth it?

"We have disseminated more than a million pieces of violence prevention public education in flyers and posters," Shapiro notes. "Approximately 80 percent have gone into the specific neighborhoods we have targeted and 20 percent have gone elsewhere in Chicago. Not only does this support our fundamental message, but just about every piece of material from us has our toll-free 800 number, where people can call us.

"That 800 number can put young people in touch with an outreach worker in their community, which is one of the most important things we deliver," Shapiro says. "There is a very high turnover rate of grassroots organizations in our neighborhoods, but CeaseFire is there every day. We provide contacts for job training, drug rehab, and other public resources. When we did focus groups with gang members and students from an alternative high school, the concept of an outreach worker who would really help you and understand some of the problems you faced in your life was one of the biggest things we could deliver."

Outreach coordinator Frank Perez explains that, unlike many programs, the people in his group will "bring the mountain to Mohammed"—bringing help to individuals who need it. They may offer their clients help in returning to school, finding a job, or simply earning a few dollars to buy a decent pair of shoes. Even before they gain their clients' trust, however, CeaseFire workers are on the scene to defuse disputes before they escalate, to hide people who are targeted for one reason or another, or to talk down a would-be killer. "We're talking to them from the public health perspective regarding the nonsense of the violence in their community," Perez says. "Ours is a carrot-or-stick approach. If you become involved in violence, then it is law enforcement's job to come in and physically remove you to make sure that you don't do this again. Our job is to prevent you from shooting that gun in the first place."

According to Perez, the most compelling outreach weapon is information, and not just the news that the violent life does not pay. Cease-Fire workers paper a target neighborhood with "Stop. Killing. People." posters, which are, according to Slutkin, "like a slap in the face." Cease-Fire posters make a statement, according to Perez. The posters show up in residential windows or on the lawn. Displaying the posters seems to imply inclusiveness—concern for the neighborhood—that belies the common urban practice of turning a blind eye. "People become—I don't know if it's cold, callous and insensitive, or just fearful—to the point that they act as if the violence doesn't exist," Perez notes. "We urge them to take a proactive approach and say, 'No, I'm not going to have people getting killed in front of my home.'"

—ᜰᜰ— CeaseFire on the Streets

Following Rapid Response procedures, the presence of CeaseFire workers in the neighborhoods makes it possible to avert escalations of warfare. Police statistics reveal that violence most commonly occurs from Thursday evening to early Sunday morning.[14] This pattern determines when CeaseFire's seventy outreach workers are on the job. Frank Perez comments, "It's not a traditional nine-to-five. It's not even a traditional work shift or workday, and it's not even a traditional kind of job, where you're expecting clients to come to you." In fact, the outreach workers want to help people out of the life that they themselves escaped, even if they have to work from sundown until sunup—which they often do.

A popular CeaseFire tactic for building community ties is a barbecue. Usually held on Friday or Saturday nights, the barbecues get started about 9 P.M. and can last until 2 in the morning. "At first, the drug dealers started moaning and groaning about us ruining their business," Perez says. "But after we started cooking and after we started delivering, they were the first ones in line." One outreach worker, Rick Jackson, usually serves as the cook. He notes, "Our idea is not just to go out and feed the neighborhood. We have a purpose: the barbecues give us a chance to pass out business cards and to talk to people in the neighborhood—to tell people what we're about—and for us to offer alternatives and resources to those who need help."

CeaseFire also makes it known through flyers that the retribution for killing someone far outweighs the temporary satisfaction of settling a score, proving one's superiority, or regaining a corner on which to sell drugs. "In the state of Illinois, when you kill someone with a gun, you're going to get at least twenty to forty years," Perez says. "If it's a gang-related homicide, you will probably see that doubled. If you get out of prison, you will be a very, very old person when you get out. So you basically sacrifice your life as well as your victim's when you pull that trigger."

Such harsh terms, plus the fact that in Illinois prisons today inmates are sometimes confined to their six-by-nine cells for twenty-three out of twenty-four hours a day, makes fiction out of the romantic stories of prison life that circulate through young gangs. Perez notes, "We say, 'Hey, you want to do that, that's fine, but check this out. Do you want to keep dealing drugs? Do you want to keep being involved in gangs? Or would you rather get your stuff together and make more money?'"

—ᴠᴠ— Outreach Workers Come Back to Their Communities

Perez and the outreach workers know whereof they speak, because most of them have been on the streets, and their credibility in the communities they serve stems from actual experience. Still, they battle such high levels of distrust that some who come from different neighborhoods must take time to gain trust in a new locale before they can be effective. "Our outreach workers come from the same lifestyle as our clients," Perez says. "We specifically hire that population to work with the gangs and the troubled individuals. There's an old Indian saying: 'You cannot judge where I've tread unless you've walked in my moccasins.'"

Outreach workers earn a modest living, but they receive health coverage, vacation, and sick time. Because they are employed through the University of Illinois system, they also are eligible to receive free tuition to any state school in Illinois. Many have taken advantage of this perk to earn bachelor's or even master's degrees. Aside from these tangible benefits, however, there is a moral and spiritual imperative. Rick Jackson, the outreach worker and cook, says, "This is my chance to give something back to the same community that I once ran through and stole from. I just wreaked havoc all through the neighborhood. Now it's my chance to strengthen it."

Jackson works with a diverse group of at-risk youngsters. Even before he joined CeaseFire, he started coaching neighborhood basketball teams when he saw that a lot of the youngsters came from single-parent homes. "They just needed a male role model, a father figure in their lives," he says. "I saw an opportunity for me to try to fill that void for a lot of them." Since he has been an outreach worker with CeaseFire, his visibility in the neighborhood has grown. Now he deals with brothers and sisters of his former clients, and the relationship contributes to his success. Even some of the young people in the neighborhood who are still dealing drugs respect him. "They have to respect me," he says. "I tell them, 'I've helped your little brother get off the corner and get into school, and I've helped your little nephew and your little cousin, and I let your other cousins play on my basketball team.'"

Recently, one of Jackson's young men garnered media attention when he entered Southern Illinois University. Shane McCoy, who once lived in a neighborhood on the other side of Chicago, was hanging out on the streets after his father and mother both turned to drugs and the family lost everything. He had dropped out of school because he was ashamed of his clothes, and when Jackson discovered the reason, he went into high gear. "I got him a job at the community center, got him back in school," he says proudly. "CeaseFire raised some money so he could go to the prom. We got a few dollars for his pocket, too. He couldn't believe it."[15]

Antonio Pickett, another outreach worker, maintains a similar passion for the program. Having spent two terms in the state penitentiary, when he first came out he began talking with eighth-graders about the hazards of street life. He often found himself arguing with kids about the new realities of what prison life was like today. "They'd say, 'What? Man, my uncle told me I get to go out to the yard and play ball and lift weights!' I said, 'No, not no more. That's over with. You are stuck in your cell.'"

Today Pickett tries to reach ex-offenders who may be in danger of returning to their previous lifestyles. "A lot of guys, they don't want to be out there selling drugs, and if somebody would give them a chance, give them a job, they wouldn't be out there sticking up stores or selling drugs. I believe this with all my heart."

Gangs have a reputation for committing violence for its own sake, but Pickett thinks that many shootings are the result of turf disputes. "If I'm selling drugs on this corner and another guy sells this end of the block, he's getting all my customers," he says. "Then there's going to be a conflict." Tio Hardiman, a community coordinator, adds that gang culture has changed in the last twenty-five years. Following the law enforcement crackdown in the 1990s after the abundance of drugs in the 1980s, large gangs began to disband, breaking up into factions and renegades. "Some were making money and some weren't, and that's what led to a lot of killings," he explains. "If you look at the statistics on homicides that were gang-related, a lot of the killings were based on old-timers trying to get their positions back." Perez believes that differences among ethnic groups are part of the problem. "Latinos are more with the machismo, more gang revenge. I don't believe that the Latinos are shooting each other that much over the drug trade. A lot of it is personal. A lot of it is easy access to a gun."

Meeting the Drug Dealers

After hearing all of the troubling descriptions of drug dealing and violence in impoverished Chicago neighborhoods, I wanted to see the streets and the drug dealers myself. Frank Perez, outreach coordinator, agreed to take me out to visit some of the neighborhoods on a Tuesday night before Thanksgiving. We were accompanied by Outreach Worker Rick Jackson.

At approximately midnight, we set out in an unmarked white Chevrolet. First, we drove down Chicago Avenue, then Augusta Avenue, through North Avenue, among many other streets. Along Chicago Avenue, which previously had been a major drug sales venue, the street was lit up as brightly as if it were daylight. High-pressure sodium lights provided illumination for the multiple video cameras with telescopic lenses that were recently installed by the city on behalf of the police department at a cost of $22,000 each. These cameras were capturing every movement along the avenue. There was not much to capture. The temperature was below freezing and few stores were open, with the exception of liquor package shops, fast-food venues, and bars. Few people were on the streets, and those who were out appeared to be rushing to get inside someplace warm.

Frank and Rick joked about how the expensive lights and cameras had displaced the drug business into the shadows off Chicago Avenue. As we worked our way further north of the city onto Fullerton Avenue, we passed a saloon, prophetically named "The Last Chance Bar." Frank and Rick pointed out that just two nights earlier, a double homicide had occurred on the sidewalk in front of the bar where we were stopped. Two local gangs, with the colorful names of the Spanish Cobras and the Imperial Gangsters, were warring. There had been five deaths by firearms in this area during the past month. A seventeen-year-old boy had been arrested for the "Last Chance" shootings. "His life is over," said Frank, shaking his head in disbelief. "In the state of Illinois, if you are over the age of 18 and kill more than one person you are eligible for the death penalty. If you don't get the death penalty, it's automatically prison for your entire natural life. He's not even wet behind the ears yet and he's never going to see daylight again."

The mood in the car was somber as we turned off the overlit avenue onto the residential side streets. The contrast in lighting was shocking—and worrisome. Other than the path of the headlights there was no illumination on these dark streets, with the exception of an occasional dim streetlight. As my eyes adjusted to the lack of light, I could see in the periphery of the headlights small groups of people, two to four, standing on roughly every third or fourth street corner. They appeared to be young men, black or Latino, and they were clearly not out to enjoy the freezing night air. I asked Frank why they didn't seem concerned about a car with a Caucasian man in the front passenger seat who was looking at them. "There are only two reasons a white guy would be in this neighborhood at this hour: either he's buying drugs or he's a cop. And you don't look like a cop. I'll show you what they think you're doing."

With that comment, Frank slowed down at the next street corner and pulled over to the curb. I rolled down the window and immediately a group of three kids, aged between thirteen and eighteen, hurried over to the car saying, "Wha cha want? Wha cha want? Rocks? Grass?" One flashed a Ziplock bag of white powder. I said something inane: "What are you guys doing out here?" As quickly as they had rushed over to the car, they receded to the shadows. If I was not a customer, I was not of interest. A similar scene was repeated twice more on other corners.

Strangely, I did not feel much sense of danger. It was late and dark in an unknown neighborhood, and uncomfortably cold, but I did not feel threatened by violence. "Well, I would not suggest that you come here by yourself," Frank said tactfully, "but you are probably not in any danger just driving around with us. Most of the shooting happens between gang members. They have much more to fear from each other than you do from them."

As Frank and Rick observed to me, the young drug dealers I was seeing probably did not carry guns themselves. "If gangs are fighting over drug territories, they might give the dealers some protection," explained Frank. "In that case, you would never see the shooter. He would be back behind a building or some bushes." Rick, who had been quiet for most of the drive, said:

"You know it is sad. They are standing out there in that cold ass weather for hours, risking arrest or worse. Most of them are minors, school dropouts. Many of them can't even read or write. The majority are from broken homes. They'll be lucky to make fifty bucks on a night like this. What else are they going to do? They can't get jobs. I want to help them just because their lives are so hopeless."

Frank responded, "Yeah, Rick, it is sad, and there are so many issues of poverty, family, education, health, employment, and so forth that need to be addressed. But I can't help a kid if he's dead. We're working on the most fundamental problem: to keep them from killing each other."

The many causes of homicide—street gang turf wars, personal disputes, drugs, domestic issues, burglary, or child abuse—make the problem more difficult to control. However, despite the varied causes of murder, CeaseFire is making a difference in some of the worst areas in Chicago: West Garfield Park experienced a 56 percent reduction in shootings after four years of CeaseFire interventions and the West Humboldt Park community had a 30 percent reduction in shootings after two years of CeaseFire activities.[16] After the first year of implementation, one of the CeaseFire beats in that district went from forty-three to fourteen shootings a year, an unprecedented reduction.[17] Overall, the CeaseFire zones of the four districts with full CeaseFire implementation have averaged a 44 percent decrease in shootings.[18] Community Coordinator Tio Hardiman notes, "We're definitely headed in the right direction. It's just a matter of the city and state opening all the way up, saying, 'OK, we've got what we need with CeaseFire. We can control violence in our communities with a unified effort that brings all the resources together.'"

Each June in Chicago, there are organized celebrations of CeaseFire Week, a time of nonstop activities in every target neighborhood, and even some neighborhoods that have yet to be added to CeaseFire's caseload. All of CeaseFire's participating partners—the churches and other social organizations—hold fairs, seminars, and fiestas to generate visibility. Hardiman observes, "It started out as CeaseFire Day. Then it became CeaseFire Weekend, and then it grew to CeaseFire Week. We don't have CeaseFire Month yet, but it's growing."

─ⅅⅅ─ The Chicago Project for Violence Prevention in the Context of Gun Violence Nationally

Some observers have noted that the results of the Chicago Project for Violence Prevention should be viewed in the context of a remarkable reduction in American homicide rates in the 1990s. That statistical phenomenon was examined in a *Scientific American* article by Richard Rosenfeld, chairman of the department of criminology and criminal justice at the University of Missouri–St. Louis.[19] Rosenfeld points out that "the national homicide rate peaked at a high of 9.8 per 100,000 in 1991, and then fell to 5.5 by 2000—a 44 percent decline." The trend lines for all crimes "began to level off by the end of the 1990s and then rose slightly from 2000 to 2001." Data for 2003 and 2004 is inconclusive.[20] His article examines various possibilities that may have affected the drop in murders, including economic trends, police crackdowns, higher incarceration rates, an apparent national decline in cocaine use, more vigorous domestic violence intervention, and more permissive "concealed carry" laws.[21] Rosenfeld concludes that no analysis of the decline provides a comprehensive explanation for the statistics.

"I would be the first person to question how much of the decline in violence can be attributed to our intervention," Slutkin notes. "There are many factors at work, but the declines in shootings directly followed our interventions, and are larger than in all comparison sites. The Chicago Project for Violence Prevention does not claim to be the only way to stop the killing. What we have demonstrated, however, is that we have a method that uses public health strategies to change community standards about violence. That does stop killings."

In his understated, nonconfrontational manner, Slutkin does not mention that the Chicago Project operated in an environment that was—and is—far more violent than the nation as a whole. In 2002, the homicide rate for Chicago was 22.3 killings per 100,000 people in the entire city—four times the national rate.[22] In the specific neighborhoods targeted by the Chicago Project, the murder rates are even higher. Moreover, the years when violence declined most markedly in Chicago Project neighborhoods occurred after the nationwide gains had already been realized. The number of shootings dropped 25 to 72 percent in the Chicago Project for Violence Prevention neighborhoods between 1999 and 2003— a time period after the national statistics had leveled out.

~ω~ CeaseFire: Sharing the Lessons Learned

From the inception of his focus on the Chicago epidemic of violence, Slutkin envisioned that the "vaccine" would be applicable in other cities, perhaps in other countries. As he outlined the success of his CeaseFire approach in speeches to professional groups around the country, numerous representatives from city commissions, police departments, and various community groups asked him for information about how to apply the same techniques in their cities. In discussions with Pauline Seitz, director of the Local Initiative Funding Partners Program, he was encouraged to write another grant application for this purpose.

"As a general policy, we do not renew Local Initiative grants," Seitz points out. "However, the Chicago Project had very well-organized findings that would be useful to other communities who are interested in replicating this model. We gave a second grant to support the Chicago Project's ability to share the lessons learned from their experiences. It is certainly not a full-scale replication. It makes sure that the Chicago Project is documented and is consolidated in a form that other communities can use to take advantage of their successes. There was definite interest on the parts of other communities in adapting this model. This second investment was made in order to capture those lessons learned and to see how they might be applied elsewhere."

As enumerated in the proposal, this new grant has five specific goals:

1. The development of CeaseFire (or CeaseFire-like) violence prevention plans with two cities

2. The development of materials for distribution to cities and states describing the CeaseFire approach, costs, benefits, and possible cost savings

3. Strengthening of data and evaluation capacity to better document project results

4. Presentations at national and other meetings of the CeaseFire approach

5. Distribution and dissemination of information on the CeaseFire approach

"As I see it, this new grant will enable us to reach three relevant outcomes," Slutkin says.

First, more U.S. cities will be able to work together to prevent violence in a civilized way. To begin, they have asked us to work with two additional cities.

We will probably work first with Baltimore and one other city that has not yet been selected. Baltimore will do its own program with its own name, but it is using many of the same ideas and same strategies that have been successful in Chicago. Second, the Local Initiative program wants us to produce some kind of operational manual for use in other communities, a sort of CeaseFire Start-up Kit. Third, we are going to look at the feasibility of creating some kind of national network, a new set of connections among cities, to prevent violence.

Sitting back in his office chair with shirtsleeves rolled up, as usual, and tie loosened, Slutkin relaxed his often serious philosophical stance and smiled broadly.

I was just thinking that next to all of the positive strides we have made in these neighborhoods, all of the killings we have been able to prevent, and all of the remarkable statistics we've chalked up, one particular CeaseFire story has touched me personally. One of our outreach workers came in last week and told me that he had been out at a late-night club in the neighborhood. It was two or three in the morning, and people had been drinking. An argument turned into an exchange of insults, and one young man pulled out a gun. Now, usually, what happens in these situations is that someone else pulls out a gun and people are killed in the resulting gunfire.

Instead, our outreach worker told me, everyone in the room just looked at the gunman as if to say: "What's wrong with you?" He looked around, embarrassed, and put the gun back in his pocket. I love that story! It shows a tangible change in community standards. It was just as if someone had lit up a cigarette in the middle of a Robert Wood Johnson Foundation board meeting. Social disapproval at its best! When I heard that story, I knew we were really making a difference, and that this could stick.

Notes

1. *Bowling for Columbine,* a documentary film written, produced, and directed by Michael Moore (a Dog Eat Dog Films Production) and released by Alliance Atlantis and United Artists, Inc.
2. Ibid.
3. WHO. *World Report on Violence and Health.* Geneva: World Health Organization, 2002.

4. Ibid.

5. Data from CDC cited by Join Together Online. (http://www.join together.org/sa/news/feattures/print/0,1856,567733,00.html).

6. Chicago Police Department, Research and Development Division. "Crime Summary—Chicago, 2003." (http://egov.cityofchicago.org/webportal/COCWebPortal/COC_EDITORIAL/03YEHomicide.pdf).

7. Ibid.

8. Chicago Police Department. "Chicago Homicides—1997." Cited in the Chicago Project for Violence Prevention grant application materials, December 3, 1998.

9. Braga, A. A., and Kennedy, D. M. "Reducing Gang Violence in Boston." In W. L. Reed and S. H. Decker (eds.), *Responding to Gangs: Evaluation and Research.* Washington, D.C.: National Institute of Justice, July 2002, p. 272.

10. Sweet, L. "Boston's Assault on Violence." *Chicago Sun Times,* March 10, 1997.

11. Leland, J. "Savior of the Streets." *Newsweek,* June 1, 1998, pp. 20–25.

12. Harden, B. "Boston's Approach to Juvenile Crime Encircles Youth, Reduces Slayings." *Washington Post,* October 23, 1997, page A3.

13. CeaseFire Web site. (http://www.ceasefirechicago.org/main_pages/clergy.html).

14. "Homicide in Chicago—December 2002." Chicago Police Department Research & Development Division, January 2003. (http://www.cityofchicago.org/CAPS).

15. Leroux, C. "Reclaiming a Neighborhood: A Life and Death Struggle for West Garfield Park." Part One of two parts. *Chicago Tribune,* November 14, 2003.

16. The Chicago Project for Violence Prevention. "Updated Results in First CeaseFire Zones." Data source: Chicago Police Department, Research and Development Division, updated by CPVP, September 22, 2003.

17. Ibid.

18. Ibid.

19. Rosenfeld, R. "The Case of the Unsolved Crime Decline." *Scientific American,* February 2004, 82–89.

20. Ibid., pp. 84, 85.

21. Rosenfeld considers the possibility that laws permitting the carrying of concealed weapons may have reduced violent crime "by making would-be offenders aware that potential victims could be armed." But he fails to note the possible deterrent effects of the Brady Bill in 1994.
22. Heinzmann, D. "Chicago Homicide Rate Still #1." *Chicago Tribune,* January 1, 2003, page 1.

Inside The Robert Wood Johnson Foundation

7

The Robert Wood Johnson Foundation: The Early Years

Joel R. Gardner and Andrew R. Harrison

Editors' Introduction

A number of chapters in the *Robert Wood Johnson Foundation Anthology* series have attempted to demystify the practice of philanthropy by examining the internal workings of The Robert Wood Johnson Foundation.[1] This chapter, written by Joel R. Gardner, who, as a consultant, has been doing an oral history of the Foundation, and Andrew R. Harrison, who serves as the Foundation's archivist, recounts the early years of The Robert Wood Johnson Foundation—from 1936 through 1975. Gardner and Harrison begin with a capsule biography of Robert Wood Johnson, who, while he was head of Johnson & Johnson, gave generously to local charities and established a small foundation for his philanthropic activities in the New Brunswick, New Jersey, area.

Johnson died in 1968, leaving just about his entire estate to the Foundation. When the will was probated, in 1972, The Robert Wood Johnson Foundation emerged as the nation's second-largest philanthropy. Gardner and Harrison capture the political circumstances into which the new and greatly expanded Foundation was born, and bring to life the early thinking about philanthropy among the first generation of Foundation staff, led by it first president, David Rogers. They discuss the ways in which early priorities and grantmaking strategies were reached between 1972 and 1975; how the concept of national programs developed; and how program evaluation and communications became integral components of The Robert Wood Johnson Foundation's approach to grantmaking.

Why focus on early history? In addition to improving our understanding of the logic of grantmaking even today at The Robert Wood Johnson Foundation, the early history can provide useful lessons for new foundations that face philosophical and organizational challenges similar to those which confronted a fledging Robert Wood Johnson Foundation more than thirty years ago. As the philosopher George Santayana wrote, "Those who cannot remember the past are condemned to repeat it."

---

1. See Hughes, R., "National Programs: Understanding The Robert Wood Johnson Foundation's Approach to Grantmaking." *To Improve Health and Health Care, Vol. VIII: The Robert Wood Johnson Foundation Anthology.* San Francisco: Jossey-Bass, 2005; Schapiro, R. "A Conversation with Steven A. Schroeder." *To Improve Health and Health Care, Vol. VI: The Robert Wood Johnson Foundation Anthology.* San Francisco: Jossey-Bass, 2003; Navarro, M., and Goodwin, P., "Program-Related Investments." *To Improve Health and Health Care, Vol. V: The Robert Wood Johnson Foundation Anthology.* San Francisco: Jossey-Bass, 2002; McGinnis, J. M., and Schroeder, S. "Expanding the Focus of The Robert Wood Johnson Foundation: Health as an Equal Partner to Health Care." *To Improve Health and Health Care 2001: The Robert Wood Johnson Foundation Anthology.* San Francisco: Jossey-Bass, 2001; Karel, F. "'Getting the Word Out': A Foundation Memoir and Personal Journey." *To Improve Health and Health Care 2001: The Robert Wood Johnson Foundation Anthology.* San Francisco: Jossey-Bass, 2001; Knickman, J. "Research as a Foundation Strategy." *To Improve Health and Health Care 2000: The Robert Wood Johnson Foundation Anthology.* San Francisco: Jossey-Bass, 2000.

—ɯ—   Ｉn a small two-story house at 142 Livingston Avenue in New Brunswick, New Jersey, The Robert Wood Johnson Foundation began its transition from a locally oriented philanthropy to the nation's leading grantmaker in the health field. Through most of the twentieth century, New Brunswick was a company town, and the company was Johnson & Johnson, one of the world's largest manufacturers of health care products. The town is also the home of Rutgers University, New Jersey's state university, and the Robert Wood Johnson medical complex of hospitals and teaching institutions. From the moment that the first Robert Wood Johnson, who founded the company with his two brothers, Mead and James, set foot in New Brunswick in 1885 and decided to establish a plant there, the town and the company have lived in symbiosis, caring and providing for each other.

It was in New Brunswick that Robert Wood Johnson married for the second time. From this marriage, he had three children, including, in 1893, Robert Wood Johnson II. Young Robert attended Rutgers Preparatory School, but when his father died in 1910, he chose to enter the family business rather than attend college. By that time, the company was providing 90 percent of cotton and gauze bandages worldwide, exported in its own steamships. By that time, too, Mead had left the company to start his own enterprise, and James succeeded to the presidency. Robert moved in with his Uncle James and worked his way up from the mill floor to the executive suite. He was appointed a director of the company at the age of twenty-one, second vice president four years later, president and general manager in 1932, and chairman of the board in 1938. Because the company was vitally concerned with the delivery of health care, he visited hospitals worldwide; he also served terms as president and chairman of Middlesex General Hospital—now the Robert Wood Johnson University Hospital—in New Brunswick.

Johnson married Elizabeth Dixon Ross, of New Brunswick, in 1916, and their wedding was the social event of the year. They moved into Bellevue, an estate in Highland Park, and their son, Robert Wood Johnson III, was born in 1920. While living in Highland Park, Johnson became involved in local politics and served a term as mayor while he was still in his twenties. His marriage broke up in 1930, and his wife and child remained at Bellevue, while he relocated with his new wife, Margaret, to Morven, in Princeton, which later became the governor's mansion. With his third wife, Evelyne, or "Evie," he moved in the 1940s to Longleat, an estate south of Princeton.[1]

From any perspective, Robert Wood Johnson was a singular individual. Though he was a firm believer in the corporate system, he promoted policies of employee support and empowerment that were radical for their time. He fought to maintain employee wages as a way of reinflating the economy during the Depression, and he developed a company credo that is a model of corporate enlightenment. During the Second World War, he was first a colonel and later a brigadier general, charged with running the Smaller War Plants Corporation, a position that the Washington columnist Drew Pearson called "the most difficult, undesirable job in government."[2] Though Johnson lacked a university education, his book, *Or Forfeit Freedom,* won the Book of the Year award from the American Political Science Association in 1948.

—w— The Johnson New Brunswick Foundation and The Robert Wood Johnson Foundation: 1936–1967

Robert Wood Johnson's first major foray into philanthropy was the Johnson New Brunswick Foundation, which was incorporated in 1936 for "charitable purposes in and about the city of New Brunswick and the County of Middlesex." The Foundation's board included his brother, J. Seward Johnson, along with prominent members of the New Brunswick community. As its first grant, made in December 1936, the Foundation donated 130 acres of land along the banks of the Raritan River in Highland Park to the County of Middlesex for use as a public park. In 1946, the Foundation gave twenty-two additional acres to the county for park space.

During the Depression and the Second World War, the Johnson New Brunswick Foundation was dormant. It had just $475 in its bank account.

After the war, however, Johnson began to build the Foundation. In 1948, he contributed two thousand shares of Johnson & Johnson stock, announced to the board of trustees that his gift represented the first of his planned annual donations to the Foundation, and arranged for the company to make a gift of $10,000.

The Foundation initiated its long-term commitment to New Brunswick's Middlesex General Hospital and St. Peter's Hospital with grants of $5,000 to each in 1948. Four years later, at Johnson's request, the Foundation removed the geographic restriction that had limited it to Middlesex County so that it could begin to fund projects and institutions throughout New Jersey while maintaining its primary focus on the New Brunswick area. In addition, the board approved a name change to The Robert Wood Johnson Foundation.

During this period, Johnson focused on strengthening the board, bringing in Johnson & Johnson executives such as Philip Hofmann, the company's president, Gustav Lienhard, its chief financial officer, and Robert Dixson, its general counsel. He passed the chairmanship of the board to Judge Klemmer Kalteissen. Norman Rosenberg, a local surgeon with ties to the company, added medical expertise. Seward Johnson left the Foundation to pursue his own philanthropic interests, but Robert Wood Johnson III served for ten years as a board member, including terms as vice president and president.

Finally, it was during this period that the Foundation's grant priorities took shape. Three areas of interest emerged: hospitals and health care; scholarship support, primarily in health care; and community service programs with a special focus on the indigent.

Approximately 65 percent of the Foundation's grant funds went to support hospitals and health care, primarily in New Brunswick. For example, the Foundation awarded $25,000 to Middlesex General Hospital for the purchase of a diagnostic x-ray machine and $27,000 to St. Peter's Hospital to buy equipment for its radiology department. Beginning in 1963, Johnson urged the Foundation to focus more attention on improving hospital management and nursing care, encouraging it to make grants to attract more people to the nursing profession and to improve the education of nurses.

The Foundation's second major interest was educational scholarships for medical, dental, nursing, and pharmaceutical students who came from low-income backgrounds. It awarded a quarter of its grant funds in the form of scholarships.

Some 10 percent of the Foundation's grant funds were directed to the third of the Foundation's priorities: assistance to community agencies and to the indigent, particularly young people. The New Brunswick YMCA and YWCA, Boys Scouts, Girls Scouts, Walter D. Matheny School (a residential facility for children with cerebral palsy), the Francis E. Parker Memorial Home in New Brunswick, the B'nai Brith Hillel Foundation, and Christ Church of New Brunswick all received donations from The Robert Wood Johnson Foundation.

—ⱳ— Transition from a Local to a National Philanthropy: 1968–1971

Robert Wood Johnson II died on January 30, 1968. At the time of his death, The Robert Wood Johnson Foundation had a net worth of more than $53 million through its ownership of Johnson & Johnson stock. Having provided for his family earlier through a series of trust funds, Robert Wood Johnson bequeathed his company stock, then valued at $300 million, to the Foundation. It took three years to probate his estate, during which time the value of the stock increased to more than a billion dollars.

Shortly after Johnson's death, the group of men closest to him began, at his request, to plan the future of his foundation. They set up a policy committee and called in experts in the field of health care to assist them in this ambitious undertaking. Even as plans for a greatly expanded Robert Wood Johnson Foundation were being drawn up, Congress was working on a tax reform act that would transform the nature of American philanthropy. Congress was moved to action by a series of events that it considered to be a flouting of the tax-exempt status enjoyed by private foundations. Members bristled at what they saw as the Ford Foundation's involvement in politics, and they were outraged by California's Irvine Foundation's and other foundations' holding enormous amounts of valuable land and other property and therefore sheltering themselves both from paying taxes and from making philanthropic grants. As a result, the 1969 Tax Reform Act included provisions that curtailed political activities on the part of foundations, prohibited the awarding of many direct grants to individuals, limited the amount of stock a foundation could hold in any one corporation to 20 percent, and, most important to Johnson's brain trust, required foundations to pay out each fiscal year an amount equal to a certain percentage of their assets (eventually settled upon at 5 percent).

Working to set up the structure of what would soon become the nation's second-largest foundation, the policy committee, overseen by the Foundation's board of trustees, concentrated on the composition of a new board and the direction that the Foundation would take. The two obvious choices for board chairman were Hofmann, the chief executive officer of Johnson & Johnson, and Lienhard, then chairman of the company's executive committee. Lienhard, closer to retirement, left the company and became chairman of the Foundation's board of trustees. The board that Lienhard led drew heavily on Johnson & Johnson executives: Dixson, Hofmann, and Lienhard, as well as Wayne Holman, Jr., and Paige L'Hommedieu. For the first time, it included an outside member of national prominence, William McChesney Martin, chairman of the Federal Reserve Board from 1951 to 1970. Rosenberg, Leonard F. Hill, a New Brunswick banker, and Judge DuBois Thompson, who replaced former board chairman Kalteissen, rounded out the roster of trustees.

In May 1971, the policy committee made two critical decisions that affected the grantmaking of The Robert Wood Johnson Foundation: first, that the Foundation's grants would have a national focus; second, that its primary purpose would be "to contribute to the advancement of health care in the United States." It recommended that the Foundation's programs and projects encompass university medical centers, hospitals, college training centers, and professional associations throughout the country while continuing to support health and social service programs in the New Brunswick area. It determined that no grants would go to support general endowments, core administrative costs, medical research, or capital facilities.

Beginning in March and concluding in December 1971, the estate of Robert Wood Johnson transferred to the Foundation 10,204,377 shares of Johnson & Johnson stock. The new Robert Wood Johnson Foundation opened its doors in December of 1971 with $1.2 billion in assets and a federal requirement that it pay out approximately $45 million in grants in 1972. By way of comparison, the earlier foundation had paid out $4.4 million in its entire thirty-four years of existence. Since under the 1969 Tax Reform Act the Foundation could no longer make the kinds of grants it had been making to individuals, it scrapped its program of direct student scholarships. Finally, despite Robert Wood Johnson's wish that the Foundation's Johnson & Johnson stock remain intact, the trustees realized that to comply with the Tax Reform Act and to meet the legal payout requirement, they would be obliged to sell some of the Foundation's shares in Johnson & Johnson.

The house on Livingston Avenue was suddenly much busier. The *New York Times* announced on December 6, 1971: "In one stroke, this philanthropic enterprise has become the second wealthiest foundation in the country, led only by the Ford Foundation." That night, apparently seduced by the lure of such riches, a burglar broke into the house. As Lawrence Foster recounts in his biography of Johnson, "The day after the story appeared, this author visited Lienhard at the Foundation office on Livingston Avenue with a draft of the annual report on grants made that year. As he approached the rear entrance of the parking lot, two workmen were rehanging the door, which had been ripped from its hinges. Lienhard was agitated. 'Some crazy jerks read in yesterday's paper that the Foundation was receiving $1.2 billion,' he said, 'and last night they broke in here trying to find it.' With a glimmer of satisfaction, he added, 'The only thing of value here was a roll of stamps.'"[3]

—⚍— Philosophy, Programs, and People: 1972–1975

Lienhard recognized that major national grantmaking, $45 million worth, was vastly beyond the scope of the board and staff that had overseen the Foundation up to that point, but he also believed that he and the board would bring fiscal expertise to the venture, thus freeing the future president to concentrate on grantmaking.

Recruiting a New President and Staff

On the day that Lienhard revealed the Foundation's bounty, he also announced the board's selection of a president. The choice was the result of
a national search for an individual whose background and reputation
would permit the Foundation to assume a leadership role quickly in health
care philanthropy. The board selected a man who seems in retrospect to
have been bred for the position.

That person was David E. Rogers. A former professor and chairman
of the Department of Medicine at the Vanderbilt University School of
Medicine, Rogers was, at the time of his hiring, dean of the medical faculty and professor of medicine at the Johns Hopkins University School
of Medicine, vice president (medicine) of the Johns Hopkins University,
and medical director of the Johns Hopkins Hospital. While at Vanderbilt, he had engaged the medical school in the struggle for integration,
and during his tenure at Johns Hopkins he oversaw the development of
health care delivery systems serving minorities and the needy in Baltimore.

Rogers was a man of vision, strength, and compassion—attributes
that he quickly imprinted on The Robert Wood Johnson Foundation.
There is a photograph of Lienhard and Rogers that hangs in the Foundation building today, showing Rogers gazing into the distance, away from
the camera lens, while Lienhard's eyes are focused squarely on him. Rogers
was to be the visionary, and Lienhard would watch him every moment.

To carry out his vision, Rogers called upon mentors, colleagues, and
protégés. His secretary of state, so to speak, was Walsh McDermott, whose
official title was special adviser to the president. McDermott, who had,
among his other accomplishments, earned an Albert Lasker Award for his
work in the drug therapy of tuberculosis, had retired as Livingston Farrand
Professor of Public Health and chairman of the Department of Public
Health at New York Hospital–Cornell Medical Center. He brought the
credibility of his medical experience to the Foundation, but his warmth
and social skills are even more strongly remembered by his colleagues from
those days.

Rogers recruited Robert Blendon, whom he had known at Johns
Hopkins. At the time Blendon joined the Foundation, he was special assistant for policy development in health and scientific affairs to the assistant

secretary and undersecretary of the federal Department of Health, Education and Welfare. Blendon's gift was creating programs out of Rogers's visions.

Rogers also reached out to the foundation world. From the Carnegie Corporation of New York, he invited Margaret Mahoney, who had worked in health care and health sciences education there. From the Commonwealth Fund, he brought in Terrance Keenan, who combined experience in health programming with a public information background, as well as nine years of work on the staff of the Ford Foundation. Together, Mahoney and Keenan provided a grounding, a sense of how things could and do get done. Both have gone on to enormous renown in the field of philanthropy, Mahoney as the first woman president of a major foundation, the Commonwealth Fund, and Keenan, who recently retired from The Robert Wood Johnson Foundation, as one of the great authorities on health and health care philanthropy.

Setting Grantmaking Priorities

The first task was to develop a perspective, not only to fulfill the mandate of the Tax Reform Act and part quickly with $45 million in grants but also to lay out a plan of attack that would enable the Foundation to have an impact on the problems confronting the American health care system. Rogers estimated that the nation would spend $80 billion on health care in 1972. The Robert Wood Johnson Foundation's payout represented less than 1 percent of that amount. He saw the Foundation as providing seed money for new programs and ideas, and hoped to arouse public consciousness by legitimizing work in neglected health fields and by motivating the public sector to assume responsibility for providing health care services. Rogers told a 1975 symposium that he and the staff agreed on a few basic guidelines: to select outcome rather than process, to limit their work to a few basic problems, to address only areas with the potential for successful human intervention, to support projects with reasonable national visibility, and to time the Foundation's efforts to coincide with a national willingness to take action.

Earlier, in the Foundation's 1972 *Annual Report,* Rogers enunciated a broader set of what might be considered founding principles. "Recognizing that The Robert Wood Johnson Foundation's resources represent the largest single source of private capital to support new efforts in the health field, we sought wide counsel to help us decide where our funds might be put to work most effectively," he wrote.

> We have studied previous foundation triumphs and failures. We have held conferences with a number of the best minds working on broad problems in health. We have had discussions with our colleagues in medicine and other health professions, and with the staffs of many of the decision makers in government who are working to develop effective legislation in health. We have also consulted with those who are users of health services, studied much of the available literature, and looked at the economic, social, and political scene in which we will operate. And we've *contemplated*—a rare privilege in our world.

Rogers recognized as well that, unlike most foundations, The Robert Wood Johnson Foundation had the resources to underwrite large-scale field tests of new ideas, not just single experiments; to pull together large numbers of groups to work on complex regional and national problems and issues; to build fields, such as primary care and emergency medical services, by surrounding core activities with supporting ones that bolster them.

Pointing to the gap between biomedical technology and the delivery of service, Rogers cited "pressing basic national problems in health," including difficulties in obtaining simple office or ambulatory medical care, especially in rural and poor urban areas; the escalating costs of medical care; qualitative inequities in the health system because of inadequate evaluation; strengthening the human caring and supportive functions of medicine; and coordination of policy planning for health and medical care. In response, Rogers continued, "the trustees and the staff have selected for our initial effort, the encouragement of institutions or individuals who are attempting to restructure the American health delivery system to make effective care more available for nonhospitalized patients." The Foundation would focus initially on three areas: improving access to medical care services for underserved Americans; improving the quality of health and medical care; and developing mechanisms for objective analysis of public policies on health.

"It is our hope that we can be effective, wise, and compassionate in interacting with those in our society seeking to better the human condition," he concluded. "We have, as an overriding belief, the conviction that human ingenuity, if given the chance, can invent practicable ways of moving toward the goals we have defined as our own—and giving that chance, in our judgment, is the appropriate and privileged role of a private philanthropic institution."

The first area of focus, improving access to medical care for underserved Americans, meant identifying, developing, and expanding the delivery of ambulatory care services. Rogers believed that the lack of a dependable primary care system represented the most pressing health problem confronting the American people. From low-income, inner-city residents and the rural poor to more affluent populations, too many Americans experienced problems in obtaining access to primary medical care. Many communities lacked adequate out-of-hospital services. Moreover, the trend toward physician specialization was leading to a shortage of generalist practitioners.

This thinking led the Foundation to establish emergency medical response systems,[4] to promote the study of generalist medicine,[5] and to support new types of health providers, such as nurse practitioners and physician assistants.[6] Increasing access to care also was the rationale for scholarship programs for minority and women medical students and medical students from rural backgrounds. Between 1972 and 1975, the Foundation provided more than $50 million to forty-eight academic medical centers to improve the delivery of, and train professionals in, ambulatory medical care.

The second priority, improving the quality of care, signified ensuring that patients received proper treatment and preventive health services. For example, the Foundation funded Georgetown University to develop a methodological tool that would measure the quality of diagnostic and follow-up care that patients received. It also attempted to improve quality by strengthening the capacity of young physicians to be better able to improve the health care system. It took over the Clinical Scholars Program from the Commonwealth Fund and the Carnegie Corporation in 1973. This program, initiated several years earlier at five medical schools—Case Western Reserve, Duke, Stanford, Johns Hopkins, and McGill—sought to enable young physicians to complement their clinical skills with training in such non-biomedical disciplines as the behavioral, management, and social sciences. The Clinical Scholars Program continues to thrive today.[7]

The third goal, improving public policy, indicated support for research into health care policies. To achieve this goal, the Foundation engaged a number of organizations to initiate centers for the study of health policy or to evaluate existing policies. It commissioned the influential *Mendenhall Report*, which confirmed the shortage of generalist physicians and indicated that 20 percent of Americans received primary care from a specialist physician; a study by the Center for Health Administration Studies at the University of Chicago that found that 24 million Americans did not have reasonable access to medical care; and a report by the Brookings Institution—carried out by Karen Davis, who later became president of the Commonwealth Fund—on the effects of government programs aimed at improving health access to medical care for the poor.

Establishing a System for Making Grants

The grantmaking process began with a small staff—Rogers, Blendon, Mahoney, Keenan, and McDermott. Their ideas, as well as ideas received from their broad contact base in the field, provided the basis for further discussion and proposals. "I wanted smart, idealistic people who were fully informed, comfortable with controversy, and who could sit around a table and disagree profoundly with one another, without taking it personally," Rogers said later. Lienhard played a vital role in the process; he could enable the easy passage of a proposal at the board level, but he also required convincing. "Walsh would describe to Gus why a project was important, and Gus would then take it to the board members," Blendon recalls. "We never lost anything at the table, but probably 50 percent of our suggestions never got that far because of Gus's opposition."

The specter of the Ford Foundation loomed over the foundation world in those days, partly because it was the nation's largest foundation and partly because of the question of staff size. Lienhard and the board wanted to avoid what they saw as Ford's bloated staff structure. They wanted a staff as lean as possible and overhead as low as possible, with a concentration on getting dollars into the field. In principle, this led to two approaches that would guide the Foundation through much of its first two decades. First, it meant that large grants were preferable to small ones; a small staff simply couldn't handle a large volume of small grants. Second, it brought about a model of grantmaking—which continues today—in which a relatively small Foundation staff was augmented by outside consultants and where administration of national programs was delegated to national program offices located outside of the Foundation.[8]

Interestingly, the notion of a small, efficient staff arose in part from a study prepared for the Ford Foundation in 1949. Anticipating the receipt of 90 percent of the shares of Ford stock, the Ford Foundation had commissioned a study to determine how it could transform itself from a local philanthropy to a national one. As reported in the *New York Times Magazine* in 1984, "One of the committee members, Don K. Price, submitted, in writing, his suggestions as to how Ford might be reorganized: keep the staff small, he wrote, and the number of grants large by turning over the programs to experts who would manage them outside the foundation."[9] Ford ignored his suggestions, but Price later shared his suggestions with Rogers, who adopted many of them. To do so, he drew on his major constituencies: hospitals, medical educators, and medical institutions large and small.

The Robert Wood Johnson Foundation started where Price left off and developed a structure for external administration that became known as the national program model. Under this model, the Foundation was able to use the services of outside program directors with specialized expertise by reimbursing their home institutions for the cost of satellite offices and staff time devoted to administering the Foundation's programs. The Clinical Scholars Program provided a prototype and an ideal test case. John Beck, former chairman of medicine at McGill, moved to San Francisco and opened an office, funded by the Foundation, from which he could administer the program. While he interacted closely with Foundation staff members, Beck managed the program, working directly with the five funded institutions.

The Emergency Medical Services Program was the first to employ a variety of features that came to characterize the national program model.[10]

It solicited proposals, using a call for proposals to announce that forty to fifty grants of up to $400,000 would be awarded. The call for proposals described what would be expected of grantees and the criteria by which applications would be evaluated by a national advisory committee of experts in the field, and the Foundation engaged the National Academy of Sciences to provide program administration.[11] Overseeing the program was assistant vice president Blair Sadler, an attorney who, with his twin brother, a physician, had helped develop Yale University's trauma program into a national resource. The program's success—as demonstrated by the federal government's picking it up—confirmed not only the potential of the National Program Office model but the efficacy of demonstration projects.

In 1972, the Foundation relocated to a plain and unimposing building in Princeton University's Forrestal Center, in a complex that had housed particle physicists and a linear accelerator. The new offices reflected Rogers' idea about how a foundation should present itself to the public. Most foundations featured lush carpeting and mahogany-paneled walls; Rogers rejected that image. He believed that lavish buildings intimidated potential grantees and siphoned off money that could go to social causes. He did not want the Foundation to appear as a place of wealth and ostentation. Staff and visitors alike had to travel up and down a cement staircase to get to the Foundation's second-floor offices, arrayed along a hallway with cinder-block walls and indoor-outdoor carpeting over a concrete floor. "We took great pride in our humble surroundings," an early staff member wryly observed.

The move from New Brunswick and the commitment to a national scope did not diminish the Foundation's commitment to support New Jersey and the community that was so important to Robert Wood Johnson himself.[12] Primarily through grants to Middlesex County Hospital and St. Peter's Hospital, but also through grants to smaller agencies such as the Society of St. Vincent de Paul of Highland Park and United Community Services of Central Jersey, the Foundation maintained its concern for the charities that it had supported for decades. Reporting to the board in May 1972, the staff recognized the Foundation's "special obligation" to the New Jersey community and proposed to address it broadly. It recognized the possibility that the state, with its dependence upon New York and Pennsylvania and its concomitant smaller medical community, might offer an opportunity to develop experimental programs. At the same time, given the paucity of other philanthropic resources in the state, it expressed a willingness to address the needs of New Brunswick and the surrounding communities.

Integrating Evaluation and Communications

Above all, the staff was writing its own scenario for the development of Foundation programming. Nowhere was this more evident than in the development of evaluation and communications programs. In both, the Foundation set out to break ground, to adopt approaches that were new to the field.

Rogers was poetic in his description of evaluation in the 1973 *Annual Report,* evoking, not inappropriately, the *Odyssey* and the *Aeneid:*

> So much for the vessels we have helped to send down to the sea this year. We have indicated some of the rocks and shoals which concern us, and have detailed some of our initial efforts to become wiser advisors. Whether the vessels we have encouraged to embark will safely make port we do not know. Perhaps in attempting to facilitate change this is all that can be done—to launch the ships and after eight to ten years look to see which ones made the trip successfully. But in our increasingly priority conscious world this passive approach would be irresponsible, and we must try to evaluate their journeys.

More prosaically, Rogers then admitted that program evaluation could not "yet be classified as a science." Still, if he was clear that the collection of data was essential to the understanding of what the Foundation was doing, he also understood that the staff would be creating its own models. "We fully recognize that we have no well-tested prescription for this exercise but we have chosen some ways to start,"[13] he said.

Rogers separated evaluations into three categories, each responding to different questions. At the simplest, the first level, the question was, "How well was the task carried out by those who conducted the program?" This, he argued, was useful internally but less so in the health professions, because it did not address the substantive issues of what the task was and what was its impact on the field.

Thus, the second level, which asked, "Did a particular program change the way individuals or institutions acted after the program was in place?" In this case, he said, the answer was useful to the community that the Foundation served, the national community of health professionals, but did not address how the Foundation carried out its programs.

At the third level, evaluations responded to the interests of "those groups and institutions which play a dominant role in the formulation of the nation's health policies and who often make the decisions regarding the flow of new resources to any social welfare field." So the questions were most focused on outcome: "Would additional expenditures of money to reproduce a particular program improve the welfare of people generally? Did it improve people's lives?"

Rogers enumerated the pitfalls as well. Change might not be immediate, and therefore not evident in the evaluation. Most programs would lack the critical mass to draw meaningful conclusions. Most institutions lacked the resources to carry out the second- and third-level evaluations. Evaluators must be sure to avoid premature evaluation, but would be better served by eight- to ten-year time frames. Finally, objective measurement was often in fact quite subjective.

Nonetheless, Rogers declared the Foundation's intention to move forward. "Perhaps with the innocence of the novitiate, we have now indicated how a start is to be made on evaluation of programs we have encouraged," he said. "Each of these efforts, and those which will follow, represent the first steps of a new foundation trying to discharge its obligations in a responsible and responsive fashion."

The same *Annual Report* lists three evaluations of Foundation programs: a three-year study of the emergency medical response program by the RAND Corporation; an evaluation of the student-aid programs by the National Planning Association; and an analysis of a program to train dentists in the care of the severely handicapped, by the Educational Testing Service.

The Foundation's evaluation function not only took root within the Foundation but also enabled academic practitioners to break new methodological ground and encouraged other foundations to hire staff members with expertise in analysis and measurement, as well as outside consultants with the skills to carry out appropriate evaluations of programs and their outcomes.

Rogers first presented to the board a proposal for a public affairs and public information program in April 1973. "As we complete fifteen months of operation," he said, the Foundation "is beginning to assume a satisfactory professional form. . . . We are well housed in comfortable quarters, we have put together a small but first-class professional staff which is viewed with respect in the foundation world and by those in medicine and the academic community. We have developed an administrative format which permits us to process grants in an orderly and well-organized fashion."

What the Foundation needed next, he continued, was to enhance its ability to communicate with the public and to "articulate the purposes which have moved us into certain sectors" by creating a public affairs and information program that was integral to the Foundation. The person selected to run the program would have a seat at the grantmaking table, Rogers proposed, and would "participate fully in the discussion of policy, the selection of areas of focus, and the consideration of proposals that we plan to support."

The person selected, Rogers continued, "should have broad experience in planning in public affairs and knowledge of organization and management of a public information staff. It would be helpful if he has had experience with academic institutions. He should have under his direction the responsibilities for building a small core staff with special skills in the communicative sciences and science writing." Frank Karel was the Foundation's choice. His background fit perfectly with Rogers' description, and he ended up transforming the way in which foundations think of communications. Karel, a journalist with a specialization in science, had moved from the *Miami Herald* to the world of health and medicine. His résumé included stops at Johns Hopkins, the National Cancer Institute, and the Commonwealth Fund.

Karel's guiding principle, which Lienhard embraced, was that the Foundation should speak through its grantees.[14] "This concept has been our communications compass for more than a quarter of a century, and has emerged as one of the core values of the Foundation," he wrote. This, along with the value placed on information by the Foundation, was underscored by including a bibliography of selected books, articles, and other information by our grantees in the 1976 *Annual Report*—a practice that has been broadened to include their work on the Web, video, data tapes, and audiovisuals, and continued to this day."[15] Over time, from these first insights, the Foundation pioneered the concept of information as a foundation asset and communications as the tool for putting this asset to work in advancing its mission, to improve health and health care.

—ɯ— **Summary**

In the *Annual Report* for 1975, Rogers summed up the work of the Foundation's first four years. "Put quite simply, helping groups to try new experiments which may contribute to better health for Americans remains our basic commitment," he wrote.

> We can assist those who are preparing people for new careers in medicine or the delivery of medical care to those not now receiving it. We can encourage the development of ways to determine whether the country has a system of acceptable quality. We can help create broader awareness of the public policy issues involved. We can attempt to stay with our programs long enough to determine their promise and to evaluate and report their impact. . . . However, improvements come slowly in any complex system, and we are but a small part of it. Nonetheless, we are encouraged by the efforts being made by the many working in the field, and we continue to be challenged by the unusual opportunity afforded us to help some of those who are busily engaged on the front lines.

His words are as true today as they were thirty-three years ago, when the leadership of The Robert Wood Johnson Foundation first contemplated the billion-dollar bequest from its founder and decided to devote its assets to improving the health and health care of all Americans.

Notes

1. Foster, L. G. *Robert Wood Johnson: The Gentleman Rebel.* State College, Pa.: Lillian Press, 1999.

2. Ibid.

3. Ibid.

4. Diehl, D. "The Emergency Medical Services Program." *To Improve Health and Health Care 2000: The Robert Wood Johnson Foundation Anthology.* San Francisco: Jossey-Bass, 2000.

5. Isaacs, S., and Knickman, J. (eds.) *Generalist Medicine and the U.S. Health System.* San Francisco: Jossey-Bass, 2004.

6. Keenan, T. "Support of Nurse Practitioners and Physician Assistants." *To Improve Health and Health Care 1998–1999: The Robert Wood Johnson Foundation Anthology.* San Francisco: Jossey-Bass, 1999.

7. Showstack, J., Anderson Rothman, A., Leviton, L. C., and Sandy, L. G. "The Robert Wood Johnson Clinical Scholars Program." *To Improve Health and Health Care, Vol. VII: The Robert Wood Johnson Foundation Anthology.* San Francisco: Jossey-Bass, 2004; Gardner, J., Krevans, J., and Mahoney, M. "A Conversation About the Clinical Scholars Program." *Medical Care,* 2002, *40*(Supp. II), 25–31.

8. For an examination of the Foundation's national program structure, see Chapter Eight in this volume.

9. Price, D. "Foundations: A Time for Review." *New York Times,* September 9, 1984.

10. Chapter Eight in this volume.

11. For an examination of the program, see Diehl, D. "The Emergency Medical Services Program." *To Improve Health and Health Care 2000: The Robert Wood Johnson Foundation Anthology.* San Francisco: Jossey-Bass, 2000.

12. For an examination of the Foundation's commitment to New Brunswick and New Jersey, see Dickson, P. "Tending Our Backyard: The Robert Wood Johnson Foundation's Grantmaking in New Jersey." *To Improve Health and Health Care, Vol. V: The Robert Wood Johnson Foundation Anthology.* San Francisco: Jossey-Bass, 2002.

13. For an examination of the Foundation's grantmaking in research and evaluation, see Knickman, J. "Research as a Foundation Strategy." *To Improve Health and Health Care 2000: The Robert Wood Johnson Foundation Anthology.* San Francisco: Jossey-Bass, 2000.

14. The principle has evolved recently to one stating, "The Foundation strives to speak with its grantees."

15. Karel, F. "Getting the Word Out: A Foundation Memoir and Personal Journey." *To Improve Health and Health Care 2001: The Robert Wood Johnson Foundation Anthology.* San Francisco: Jossey-Bass, 2001.

8

National Programs: Understanding The Robert Wood Johnson Foundation's Approach to Grantmaking

Robert G. Hughes

Editors' Introduction

When The Robert Wood Johnson Foundation became a national philanthropy, in 1972, it had to come up quickly with a way to distribute millions of dollars a year to its grantees. The national program model that the Foundation staff developed in the early years—in which the management of a related group of grants is delegated to an outside organization—has served as the Foundation's principal grant management mechanism for more than thirty years. It has been particularly well suited to demonstration programs where an approach to a problem, or variations

Thanks to the many people who have shared their understanding of national programs with me. In particular, Calvin Bland, Peter Goodwin, Ruby Hearn, Rona Henry, Frank Karel, Terry Keenan, Julia Lear, Janice Opalski, and Warren Wood helped develop my understanding of national programs. Bob Blendon, who by all accounts was a principal architect of the national program model, was especially helpful in articulating the impact of the Ford Foundation Report on the Foundation's thinking early on. Special thanks to Andrew Harrison for assistance in locating Foundation historical material. Of course, I remain ultimately responsible for the ideas expressed in this chapter.

of an approach, are tested at a number of different locations. Delegating program management has also created opportunities for talented professionals working outside the Foundation to assume leadership roles on specific aspects of health and health care.

In this chapter, Robert G. Hughes, the chief learning officer at The Robert Wood Johnson Foundation, examines the historical roots of the national program model, explores the factors that led the Foundation to adopt it, discusses the ways in which the model has evolved, and analyzes the issues facing the Foundation as it reexamines its options for making and managing grants. Hughes also assesses the strengths and the weaknesses of this approach to grant management, particularly in the context of the tension between maintaining a small program staff and exercising careful oversight of programs.

The Robert Wood Johnson Foundation recently established a new office of national program affairs headed by its former treasurer, Peter Goodwin. The creation of this office signals an interest in updating and reconsidering the Foundation's approach to managing national programs. Given a total annual budget of nearly $117 million a year for the staffing and administration of more than eighty different National Program Offices, finding ways to manage national programs more effectively and efficiently is emerging as an important Foundation priority.

—ᴡ— In 1972, six people sat around a lunch table down the hall from rented offices at the former site of a nuclear accelerator in Plainsboro, New Jersey. Their wide-ranging lunchtime discussions touched on the many ways philanthropy could help improve health care and, ultimately, the health of the population. There were many such discussions among that group, all of whom were early staff members of The Robert Wood Johnson Foundation. The ideas emerging from these sessions, along with those of the board of trustees, numerous advisers, and health care experts from around the country, shaped the basic direction of the Foundation during its formative years. Outside observers and potential grantees were most interested in what the Foundation would choose as program areas and the problems and issues that the Foundation would try to address in its grantmaking.[1] But the Foundation trustees and staff members had another question to answer—a more mundane one in some ways— how to distribute the Foundation's substantial funds responsibly.

When the Foundation received the proceeds from the estate of Robert Wood Johnson, it became the nation's second-largest philanthropy in the country overnight, with assets of more than $1 billion. The Foundation needed to award about $45 million per year. Its challenge was to make grants that would reflect Robert Wood Johnson's values and further the board's vision for the Foundation. At the heart of the challenge was a practical administrative problem: reconciling the desire to review each grant proposal carefully and to monitor the work of each grantee with the desire to minimize the costs of this review and oversight. Underlying the practical problem were issues of control and delegation; the roles of the board, the staff, and the grantees; and how the grantmaking mechanisms adopted would affect the Foundation's standing with its constituents.

Representing a practical compromise between the Foundation's desire to maintain a relatively small staff and minimal bureaucracy and its need to monitor programs scrupulously, a mechanism called the national program emerged as the Foundation's principal vehicle for grantmaking. In a national program, an organization outside the Foundation would oversee a set of grants related to a particular field. Experts in fields that were the focus of national programs would not have to be hired by the Foundation as employees but would remain in their home institutions, devoting a percentage of their time to the program. When the program ended, they would simply resume their former duties.

Throughout the Foundation's thirty-three-year history as a national philanthropy, national programs have been used to distribute the bulk of the Foundation's grants. Approximately 65 percent of the more than $5 billion in grants since 1972 has been awarded via 219 national programs.

—⁜— What Is a National Program?

While no two national programs appear exactly alike, most of them have six basic characteristics in common:

1. *Foundation staff members and national experts, sometimes working with a consultant not on the Foundation's staff, develop a program designed either to address a problem of national scope or to take a promising model or idea that has received limited exposure and subject it to broader testing.* Such programs typically emerge over a year or two through a process of meetings, reviews, consultations, and revisions that involve Foundation staff members, outside experts, and practitioners from the field. During this developmental period, a program's purpose is refined, and many of its basic features—such as desired outcomes, number of grantees, grantee activities, eligibility criteria for applicant organizations, amount of grants, and duration of the program—are discussed and drafted.

2. *A call for proposals, or CFP, is distributed to potential applicants and others in the field.* The CFP defines the problems or the issues central to the program and describes the program's purpose; the desired outcomes; eligibility criteria for applicants; how the funds may be used; the criteria and the process for selecting grantees, grant amounts, and duration; and the number of grants or sites to be funded. In addition, a CFP includes the application and selection timetable, and identifies the individuals and the organizations responsible for management, oversight, and evaluation

of the program. CFPs are distributed after the board of trustees authorizes a program. Substantial changes in the program—such as major revisions of its purposes or activities, an extension of its duration, and additional funding—must be approved by the board.

3. *Grantees are selected through a national competitive process, and any organization that meets the program's eligibility criteria can apply.* The selection of program sites—grantees under the program—from among the applicants is done by a national advisory committee, or NAC, made up of experts from a variety of areas related to the program. The NAC members review the written proposals, conduct site visits at selected applicant institutions, and recommend applicants for funding to the Foundation. The NAC is typically asked to meet periodically throughout the life of the program, providing advice and counsel to the national director of the program as well as monitoring and reporting on the progress of the program to the Foundation.

4. *The Foundation establishes a National Program Office, or NPO, external to the Foundation.* Usually based at a university or other nonprofit organization, an NPO organizes the grantee selection process and the work of the national advisory committee. After grantees are selected by the Foundation and funds are awarded, an NPO monitors the work carried out under the grant, provides technical assistance to the program sites, and facilitates collaboration and the sharing of information—through annual meetings, for instance. In most cases, NPOs are expected to provide leadership to the field. A distinctive feature of national programs, NPOs are the Foundation's solution to the basic administrative dilemma of wanting knowledgeable and thorough program oversight while at the same time avoiding an unduly large home-office staff.

5. *Formal program evaluations, intended to help the Foundation and the field learn from national programs, are conducted by organizations independent of the Foundation, the NPO, and the sites funded under the program.* Selected by a competitive process, the evaluators use social science and anthropological and other widely accepted techniques to assess program impact, effectiveness, implementation, and other aspects of performance. Evaluators are expected to produce final reports meeting the

standards of appropriate scientific and professional journals, and are encouraged to submit their reports for publication in peer-reviewed and other journals and to present their findings at professional meetings.

6. *Information about the programs is shared with the field through communications activities.* National programs are supposed to have an impact beyond the sites themselves, and publicity about a program's activities and results is essential if this is to occur. Similarly, communications support, often from a program's inception, is needed if the activities of participating sites are to continue after the grant ends. These communications functions may be carried out by the NPO staff, by Foundation staff members, by outside consultants, or by a combination of these options.

These six characteristics make up the basic framework of the Foundation's national program model. A brief overview of more than eighty national programs operating in 2003 conveys the scale and the considerable range within this general model: the number of sites in a national program ranges from fewer than ten to several hundred, with an average of about twenty-five. Grants to program sites vary from tens of thousands to millions of dollars; the average is $300,000.

These numbers indicate the flexibility that the national program mechanism allows. Indeed, highlighting the common features of national programs may convey the idea that national program structures are straightforward and are more similar to one another than different. In fact, however, national programs vary in size and scope, and the six components are often modified to reflect a particular program's needs.

—ɯ— Philanthropy and The Robert Wood Johnson Foundation in 1972

How did The Robert Wood Johnson Foundation come to develop national programs with these six basic characteristics as its principal grant-making approach? The answer begins in 1972, when the Foundation received the endowment from the estate of Robert Wood Johnson. At that time, all of the ten largest foundations had been established for at least twenty years, and it would be twenty years more until the next cluster of new large foundations came along. The Robert Wood Johnson Foundation might have relied on established foundations as models, but in the 1960s a series of congressional hearings critical of big philanthropies culminated in 1969 legislation establishing stricter laws to govern foundations. The hearings raised concerns about the political influence of foundations—from supporting voter-registration drives to being refuges for governmental officials who had left office. These hearings and the resulting legislation received considerable public attention, and thus sensitized Robert Wood Johnson Foundation officials to the risks that had brought controversy to other large foundations.[2]

The Foundation's initial focus on health care set it apart from other large foundations (which made grants in multiple areas, such as education, economic development, the arts, poverty, and the environment) and limited its substantive area of grantmaking. Funding only in the United States further concentrated the Foundation's grantmaking; many other large foundations made grants for international projects. Thus, The Robert Wood Johnson Foundation's domestic health care mission helped set the stage for the development of a distinctive grantmaking approach.

While the health care mission conveyed clearly what would not be funded, the task of selecting from the many worthwhile topics and problems within health care remained. By 1972, the country had come to rely on government for basic biomedical research (via the National Institutes of Health, which began to burgeon in the 1960s) and for health care financing for the elderly and the poor (via Medicare and Medicaid, begun in 1965). Counterparts to notable philanthropic health successes earlier in the century—such as Rockefeller's hookworm eradication in the South and the development of a yellow fever vaccine—would not be matched in this new era of huge government funding. Rather, a new, more selective focus within health care was needed to avoid duplication with governmental activities and to leverage the Foundation's grantmaking.[3]

The widely expected passage of national health insurance legislation during the Nixon administration provided a framework. As the very first Foundation staff paper stated, "the reconstitution of the Robert Wood Johnson Foundation as a national philanthropic organization comes at a unique point in American history. The nation has reached the culmination of a forty-year debate over the need to eliminate economic barriers to access to personal health services. Thus, within three years, we believe we are likely to see the enactment of some form of national health insurance program." National health insurance would address financing, but it also would highlight the health care system's inability to deliver care, especially primary care, for the entire population. This led the Foundation to choose improving access to primary care as one of its three initial goals.[4] The Foundation planned to reach this goal in part by demonstrating innovative models of service delivery that the federal government could adopt for the anticipated new national health care financing system. Demonstration projects in multiple locations fit well with the grantmaking mechanism of national programs.

These factors influenced the Foundation's initial grantmaking approach, but the biggest influence was a 1949 report prepared for the Ford Foundation as it coped with a similar stage in its organizational history. As Robert Wood Johnson Foundation officials talked with those at other large foundations to learn how they had structured their grantmaking, this report emerged as a seminal document. The *Report of the Study for the Ford Foundation on Policy and Program* was a wide-ranging document, the culmination of an effort that included twenty-two other special and individual reports.[5] It was prepared in anticipation of the Ford Foundation's receiving large endowments from the estates of Henry Ford and Edsel Ford. One section of the report, "The Administration of the Program," was particularly relevant for The Robert Wood Johnson Foundation, because it presented a "suggested pattern of operations"—grantmaking approaches—for the Ford Foundation. The practical issues associated with granting large sums of money are seldom the topic of thoughtful analysis, so this was an unusual document.

The report's authors highlighted two ideas that guided their thinking in producing recommendations: maintaining flexibility of operations and giving trustees the best opportunity to guide the program in a general way. These ideas were reflected in recommendations for the types of institutions the Ford Foundation should work with and the roles of the trustees and the staff. First, the report recommended that the Ford Foundation not become involved in direct program operations but, rather, work through other organizations: These so-called intermediary organizations, which could be existing institutions such as universities or new entities established specifically to further the program's purpose, "would be free to administer the fund and make grants from it quite independently of the Foundation."

According to the Ford report, the role of the trustees was to set the general direction and to address policy questions—not to review individual grant proposals. The report pointed out that for the trustees to carry out their responsibility, they should not get involved in the detailed operations of the foundation. In keeping with the independence of intermediary organizations, the report stated, "Once a grant is given for a project, the Foundation officer should not attempt to control it. On the contrary, he should make every effort to leave full responsibility in the hands of the man in charge of the project and if asked for advice he should give it only with restraint and detachment." The staff and the trustees could review a body of work when an intermediary's term was done, with an eye toward renewal of work in that topical area, or not, depending on the merits. The report recommended recruiting a staff with a broad range of interests so that expertise in one area did not become a liability when the Foundation moved on to other areas.

In sum, the report to the Ford Foundation envisioned a structure in which the trustees would operate at a policy level (by examining broad issues, setting the foundation's direction, and judging performance); the staff would be more involved in implementation but would have sufficient detachment to make critical judgments and recommendations about the grantmaking directions and to assess the performance of intermediary organizations; and intermediaries would do most of the operational work of making and monitoring individual grants.

Many of the basic features of this proposed structure appealed to The Robert Wood Johnson Foundation. Both the board and the early staff members wanted to maintain flexibility and did not want to develop a large staff. On the other hand, in 1972 there were strong influences on The Robert Wood Johnson Foundation to maintain tight oversight of future grantees. These influences included the public scrutiny of philanthropy in general and of a new large foundation in particular; the values of Robert Wood Johnson; and the culture of Johnson & Johnson, from whose ranks most of the early board members came, which called for careful attention to detail and for close monitoring of budgets. So while the proposed Ford Foundation model of operations was appealing, the extent to which it ceded responsibility to intermediaries was not compatible with the heritage of the founder and the company whose stock was the source of the Foundation's endowment. It also ran against the environment of the time, which culminated in the 1969 Tax Reform Act—the act that required greater accountability and oversight on the part of private foundations.

As a result of these tensions—maintaining flexibility versus exercising control; delegating responsibility versus maintaining careful oversight; utilizing the expertise of leaders in the field versus delegating too much authority over Foundation resources—the Foundation adopted a variation on the approach recommended by the Ford Foundation report. It built on the idea of using intermediaries, but the design features were developed over time through the practical work of grantmaking.

—⚬⚬— Initial National Programs

Every year from 1972 to 1978, the Foundation initiated two to four programs that, in retrospect, can be recognized as national programs. The 1973 *Annual Report* noted that two external organizations, the National Academy of Sciences and the American Fund for Dental Education, were responsible for administering programs to establish emergency medical systems and dental care for the handicapped, respectively. The term "national program" was used only to describe the Clinical Scholars Program, which was administered by an outside director on the faculty of the University of California, San Francisco, although the use of the term was not intended at the time to denote a set of specific program characteristics. The 1974 *Annual Report* stated that the Foundation had "launched seven national programs of differing size and complexity," emphasizing several structural features: they were invitational, open to "a wider group than commonly receive foundation assistance," and used outside professional groups for formulation and design. It also noted, "In an effort to keep our internal staff small, an outside organization has often been asked to assume responsibilities for implementation and day-to-day management." The 1975 *Annual Report* listed eight national programs and contained a chart showing the amount and percentage of grants that went to these programs. It captured this constellation of characteristics in a summary description: "Foundation-initiated invitational programs—our national programs."

How did the national program model become established in just a few years? Several early programs incorporated design features that became part of the Foundation's national program model. The board authorized the first national program, for scholarship funds at American medical and osteopathic schools, at a level of $10 million. The Association of American Medical Colleges, or AAMC, administered this program for $10,000 a year, foreshadowing the role that would become a National Program Office. "The Association has ready access to the information required, an experienced statistical staff, and first-rate management," a staff paper noted at the time. "Thus the Foundation can undertake a program involving the administration of 115 grants with minimal expenditure of the time of its own limited staff."

The Emergency Medical Services Program was the first to include a competitive call for proposals, or CFP. The CFP told the field the grant amounts ($400,000) and the number to be awarded (forty to fifty), who could apply, and the selection criteria a national advisory committee of experts from the field would use to choose grantees. The Foundation awarded a separate $300,000 grant to the National Academy of Sciences to administer the program, which included managing the advisory committee, site visits, and evaluation. In choosing an outside organization, "the Foundation is following a policy of decentralizing the administration of single-purpose national grantmaking programs of limited time duration," thus augmenting the responsibilities of an intermediary beyond what the AAMC had done in administering the student aid program.

Quickly on the heels of the Emergency Medical Services national program, three new demonstration programs—Dental Training for Care of the Handicapped, the Community Hospital–Medical Staff Group Practices Program, and the Regionalized Perinatal Care Program—reinforced the basic design features: a program developed by staff and senior program consultants, a widely publicized CFP, and the use of expert national advisory committees to review proposals and conduct site visits. However, the Foundation did not use the national program model only for demonstrations. Two programs the Foundation started funding in 1973—the Clinical Scholars Program and the Health Policy Fellows Program—illustrated the versatility of the national program model by using it for initiatives supporting leadership training for health professionals. These programs supported individuals rather than organizations providing services, but they used the basic design structure, including an external National Program Office and a national advisory committee to review applicants. The Clinical Scholars Program, which had been picked up from the Commonwealth Fund and the Carnegie Corporation of New York, already had projects at five universities, so the existing multisite idea was consistent with the developing national program model.

Evaluation has been a critical component of the national program model. But the model didn't create the institutional commitment; rather, the commitment to assess programs existed from the time the Foundation became a national philanthropy, and it was incorporated into the model. A 1973 staff paper noted, "We envision a Foundation which supports demonstration programs as proposed solutions to health problems, which provides explicit mechanisms for evaluating these demonstrations, and through such processes, attempts to resolve those health problems that arise." The earliest national programs had evaluations built in, and as the model evolved, it became the norm for the Foundation to make a grant to an outside organization—not the NPO—for the purpose of evaluating a national program.

A final national program design element—communications—was prompted by staff thinking about what, if anything, the Foundation should do as a national program neared its conclusion. As the EMS program was ending, staff members examined options for the sustainability of existing program sites and the replication of the tested model in other sites. Replication, in particular, was a conceptual underpinning of the national program model when it was used for service demonstrations. The Foundation added communications to the national program design for two purposes: "to ensure that new options emerging from our programs gain sufficient visibility to receive appropriate consideration nationally" and "to share the knowledge, experience, and insights gained in our programs with those who decide to accept the new option and begin the process of replication."

The application of communications to foster sustainability came later. Other types of technical assistance, for grantees as well as for similar programs throughout the country, were prompted in order to help promote replication and foster the sustainability of funded projects. While technical assistance was typically provided by the National Program Office, other organizations were also used. "We have found that companion efforts can maximize the success of a national program," a 1974 staff paper noted. "For example, as part of the EMS program administered by the National Academy of Sciences organization, the Foundation and the American Medical Association are co-sponsoring four workshops open to all program applicants."

The Foundation's initial grantmaking experience with unsolicited proposals from the field reinforced the value of inviting organizations to compete for grants through national programs. David Rogers, the Foundation's first president, captured this aspect of national programs in the 1974 *Annual Report.* After noting that the Foundation had made many single grants to organizations that sought help for projects within the Foundation's areas of interest, he wrote that this kind of grantmaking

> made us recognize that in a number of instances, multiple groups or institutions simultaneously wish to attack the same problem in different regions, using their particular resources, or their particular circumstances, in different, yet quite similar ways. This kind of broadly voiced interest in a particular problem has led us to develop a series of one-time grants nationally announced, and awarded in a number of institutions participating in a broader national effort directed at a particular need. These are foundation-initiated programs in areas where a certain critical level of activity seems needed to gain experience with, or demonstrate the worth of, a particular approach.

—᠉— Early Assessment of the National Program Approach

Aware that its behavior was closely scrutinized by Congress, staff members of the young Robert Wood Johnson Foundation thought carefully about how they did their grantmaking. Around the time that the idea of a national program coalesced, a staff paper entitled "National Competitive Grant Programs" examined the advantages and the disadvantages of such programs.

Heading the list of advantages was the fact that programs were "open to all." Early on, the Foundation decided on a process open to a wide variety of applicants. "We made these decisions with the belief that the difficulties many groups have obtaining information about and access to grants has been the Achilles' heel of foundations, and it has caused many to feel that foundations are elitist or arbitrary in their awards," David Rogers and two of his senior Foundation colleagues wrote in 1983. "Because of unfamiliarity with foundations in general, or a lack of understanding of our mission in particular, many who might make important contributions to the improvement of health affairs might not find their way to us unless we make a special effort to reach out to a broad constituency."[6] The Foundation valued the fairness and the benefits of a competitive process based on expert judgments and clear criteria. This process was an antidote to the reality and the perception that philanthropy was an insider's game in which who you knew was more important than demonstrated merit or promise. It also reduced the risk that The Robert Wood Johnson Foundation would be criticized for perceived political bias in its grantmaking practices.

This open competition was compatible with the emphasis on the "national" in national program. For board members, a national perspective was important as a way of distinguishing the post-1972 Foundation from the earlier Robert Wood Johnson Foundation, with its focus on central New Jersey. In fact, The Robert Wood Johnson Foundation's first letter to potential applicants said that it would concentrate on programs that were "fully national in scope" and that it would support those that showed "promise of having significant regional and national impact."[7]

A national perspective was also important in its geographic sense. Annual reports typically included a chart showing percentage of grants, dollars, and American population for each region of the country to demonstrate that the Foundation's activities were widely distributed (and, implicitly, that they were not bundled locally as a result of favoritism). An anecdote, perhaps apocryphal, indicates how valuable this distribution was to Gustav Lienhard, chairman of the board from 1972 to 1985. A conference room had a United States map displayed with pins to indicate the location of early Foundation grants. After looking at this map one day and seeing a concentration of pins in the Northeast, Lienhard said, "Scatter the pins!"—an admonition that has shaped Foundation grantmaking ever since. This approach, which supported a large number of local projects nationwide, also satisfied board members who valued a traditional charity program that helped people, while accommodating those who valued the analysis and evaluation activities that contributed to useful knowledge about program effectiveness.

Moreover, the national program model was valued for its efficiency. "The development of a national program is a time-consuming process, but probably modest in contrast to the considerable time and resources that are expended by the Foundation staff in developing a single proposal," an early staff paper noted.

While a national program approach using a competitive grant application process had great advantages for the fledgling Foundation, it did not answer the question of whether programs should be overseen from inside or outside the Foundation—the very question raised by the 1949 report to the Ford Foundation. An analysis of the pros and cons of using external National Program Offices to administer grants identified the several advantages and disadvantages, as shown in Table 8.1.

The list suggests the underlying issues at play. The desire to keep the staff small was pitted against the risk of losing control over program administration. Inconsistencies between the Foundation's view of a program and a partner organization's view could create conflicts. The division of responsibility between the Foundation and an outside institution was ambiguous. But one design feature not mentioned was unambiguous—who controlled the money, and that was the Foundation. The outside institution received its own grant, of course, but the program sites were funded directly by the Foundation, not through the partner organization. Accordingly, advice from national advisory committees about which applicants to fund went to the Foundation, not to the National Program Office. This role for NPOs was considerably less than the intermediary role recommended in the Ford Foundation report. The decision to retain

Table 8.1   Advantages and Disadvantages of
Using External Program Offices to Administer Grants

Advantages	Disadvantages
Keeps headquarters staff small	Less control over programs
Permits Foundation staff to plan longer range	If poorly administered by partner, considerable Princeton staff time required
Removes the Foundation from basic selection process—reduces criticism and places pressure directly on Princeton staff	Partner organization may have different perception of its role from that of the Foundation
Involves a major organization as a partner with the Foundation—which should enhance the Foundation's prestige	Key executive officer of partner organization may have different perception of his role than the Foundation
Educational for the Foundation—partner organization will learn things from the field that the staff would not	Complicated to administer

fiscal oversight by the Foundation was a critical one that has shaped the roles, responsibilities, and relationships of Foundation staff members, NPOs, and program grantees ever since.

In addition to the substantive and administrative issues, the emergence of national programs had a political dimension. The national program model afforded considerable credibility to a new foundation. As a new entity, The Robert Wood Johnson Foundation had an uncertain standing in philanthropy and in health care. The Foundation gained immediate prestige when the board of trustees selected David Rogers, dean of the Johns Hopkins School of Medicine, as the Foundation's president. The recruitment of experienced staff members from other foundations also gave the Foundation credibility in the philanthropic community. Within the health care community, the national program model helped the young Foundation establish credibility because it engaged health care experts in all facets of the program, especially as leaders of National Program Offices, as members of national advisory committees, and as senior program consultants.

Many National Program Offices and grantees were also part of the Foundation's primary constituency—academic health centers and medical schools in particular. Indeed, in the Foundation's first three years, 65 percent of the funds went to academic centers.[8] The national program model was compatible with the way academic health centers operated. They relied extensively on grants; faculties cooperated across institutions in multisite clinical trials and other research projects; they were accustomed to a competitive peer-review system of grant selection; and the intermingling of practice with science in medicine paralleled the combination of demonstration with evaluation in Foundation programs.

—ɰ— Evolution of National Programs

As a grantmaking vehicle, the national program mechanism has been remarkably consistent since it was established in the mid-1970s. The basic structure has become institutionalized within The Robert Wood Johnson Foundation. A 2003 national program such as Active Living by Design, which integrates physical activity into community planning efforts, looks, in its grantmaking structure, remarkably similar to the Emergency Medical Systems Program, launched thirty years earlier. But this consistency in basic structure should not obscure two important aspects of the evolution of national programs: the increasing number of programs and the variations within the basic model.

The increasing number of national programs—the Foundation had more than eighty in 2004—was driven by five interrelated factors: growth in Foundation assets and staff, staff incentives, increased diversity of funding areas, decreased size of programs, and the continuation of existing programs, even as new ones were added. As Foundation assets have grown over the years, new staff members have been hired to oversee the concomitant increase in grants. For Foundation staff members, developing a national program became a hallmark accomplishment; it was one of the few ways a program officer could gain recognition within the Foundation and in the field generally. Over the past thirty-plus years, the Foundation has entered new substantive areas—tobacco control and end-of-life care, for instance—and this has required new programs with new institutions and people. The pressures for new programs led ineluctably to smaller programs, although this was not obvious because the nominal size of national programs remained fairly constant, at around $10 million. But $10 million in 1973 dollars was approximately $40 million in 2003, so in real dollars the programs became smaller. Finally, as existing programs were renewed while new programs were developed, the net result was an increasing number of active programs.

The second important aspect of the evolution of national programs was the variation among NPOs.

- The types of organizations used as NPOs have been diverse: professional associations, medical care delivery organizations, independent nonprofit entities, and policy institutes joined academic institutions as NPOs.

- The staffing of NPOs became less standard—some had full-time program directors, communications staff, and financial monitoring staff; deputy directors, who formerly were responsible for standard administrative functions, assumed more prominence, and in some cases were virtually indistinguishable from the directors in their substantive contributions to the field.

- NPOs have played a variety of roles. Some NPOs, such as the Center for Health and Health Care in Schools at George Washington University and Join Together, are resource centers that provide technical assistance to organizations in their fields across the country. The Center for Prevention Research at the University of Kentucky, the NPO for the Research Network on the Etiology of Tobacco Dependence, administers a network program structure that fosters intellectual work among grantees. Several NPOs experimented with new grantmaking roles—for example, by administering special grant funds for projects to take advantage of fast-breaking opportunities. A few NPOs, such as the Center for Health Care Strategies, which is the NPO for the Medicaid Managed Care Program, took on direct responsibility for grantee selection under the program, moving closer to a more independent intermediary role.

The evolution of national program structures is reflected in their nomenclature and brief descriptions found in the Foundation's annual reports. Table 8.2 lists these for 1973–2002.

Initially, only the names and the degrees of the senior program consultants were listed; the job title changed to "program director" in 1988. This original listing emphasized a person rather than an organization, and that person was considered an expert with a consulting relationship to the Foundation (even when the consultant's home institution had a grant to administer the program). Defining that person as a consultant reinforced the Foundation's authority over the program. The shift to "program director" in 1993 connoted that the program's leader shared responsibility for the program with the Foundation, an idea that was strengthened by adding "National Program Office" to the heading. Contact information for the NPO was included for the first time, along with an explanation that stated, "Most of these programs are managed by institutions outside the Foundation." The most recent change, in the 2001 *Annual Report,* emphasized the growing heterogeneity of program structures and associated strategies by referring to intermediary organizations as "National Program Offices and Resource Centers."

The quantity and the variety of national programs have produced administrative challenges for the Foundation. The large number of small

Table 8.2 National Programs: 1973–2002

Date	Title	Information	No. of NPs
1973–1987	Senior Program Consultants	Name, degree	4–24
1988–1992	Program Directors	Name, degree	24–37
1993–2000	National Program Offices and National Program Directors	Program name Director's name Organization and address	37–80
2001–2003	National Program Offices and Resource Centers	Program name Organization and address Web site address Director's name and e-mail address	80

programs increased the staff needed to develop, monitor, and learn from individual programs. The variety of program models has resulted in ambiguity and duplication of roles between Foundation staff and NPO staff. This is costly and erodes the benefits of delegation to outside offices. Growing recognition of these issues led to an October 2003 staff paper that reviewed the Foundation's use of NPOs. Based on an internal study of National Program Offices as a vehicle for grantmaking and grant management, the staff paper found that using so many different NPOs to perform common functions led to "inefficiencies." The paper focused on the same question raised in the report to the Ford Foundation's board back in 1949—which functions should be performed internally by the Foundation's staff and which should be delegated to outside organizations.

The answers are still not in, and The Robert Wood Johnson Foundation is still looking for the appropriate balance between in-house and external program management. In the current environment, where nonprofit organizations must be more accountable, foundations must devote appropriate resources not only to making grants but also to monitoring programs, assessing performance, learning what works, and communicating with the field and the public. To meet the challenges, the Foundation needs to identify clearly the variety of program models it will use, so that staff and grantees alike understand their roles in the program model they work within. Equally important, to increase the overall effectiveness of its programs, the Foundation needs to learn how different program models relate to the impact of the programs.

—w— Conclusions

National programs as a grantmaking approach emerged as a compromise between the delegation of grantmaking responsibility to an intermediary organization and retaining the responsibility within the Foundation. The benefits of delegation (avoiding a foundation bureaucracy, flexibility, use of outside experts, and a staff focus on learning from investments rather than spending time on the mechanics of retail grantmaking) were at odds with the benefits of maintaining direct control over the use of Foundation grants (specifying program goals and activities, understanding grantees' work, and holding grantees accountable financially and programmatically). The hybrid that developed had the benefits of both approaches, but it also had their disadvantages. Almost inevitably, the insistence on control and detailed plans for the use of grant funds required staff growth within the Foundation and an emphasis on grantmaking over learning about the results of multiple investments in a program area. At the same time, partial delegation of program responsibilities has resulted in inefficiencies and confusion about the relative roles of Foundation and National Program Office staff. The future challenge for national program design is to use grantmaking approaches that exploit the advantages and minimize the disadvantages of both approaches.

Notes

1. Farber M., "Suddenly Wealthy Johnson Foundation Maps Plans." *New York Times,* May 12, 1972.
2. Chapter Seven in this volume.
3. Blendon, R. "The Changing Role of Private Philanthropy in Health Affairs." *New England Journal of Medicine,* 1975, *292,* 946–950.
4. The other two initial goals were improving the quality of health and medical care and developing mechanisms for objective analysis of public policies in health. *The Robert Wood Johnson Foundation Annual Report.* Princeton, N.J., 1972.
5. Study Committee (H. R. Gaither, Jr., Chairman). "Report of the Study for the Ford Foundation on Policy and Program." Ford Foundation, November 1949.
6. Blendon, R., Aiken, L., and Rogers, D. "Improving Health and Medical Care in the United States: A Foundation's Early Experience." *Journal of Ambulatory Care Management,* November 1983, 1–11.
7. "Information on The Robert Wood Johnson Foundation." Informational letter to all applicants, September 25, 1972.
8. "Chartbook of Expenditures 1972–1974." The Robert Wood Johnson Foundation, Princeton, N.J., 1975.

–ᴠᴠ–Index

A

AAMC (Association of American Medical
Colleges), 187
Active Living by Design, 193
Addressing Tobacco in Managed Care,
19–20, 22
"The Administration of the Program" (*Report
of the Study for the Ford Foundation*), 184
Adults Don't Crawl campaign (NU Direc-
tions), 60
Advocacy Institute, 21, 26
Agency for Health Care Policy and Research,
18
Agency for Healthcare Research and Quality,
18
Aguirre-Molina, M., 55, 102, 117
Aiken, L., 76, 79
Albert Lasker Award, 163
Alcohol use: consequences of underage,
50–51; unappreciated consequences of
binge, 51–53. *See also* Youth drinking
Altman, D., 21–22
AMA (American Medical Association), 13,
33, 38, 43, 46, 54
American Association of Colleges of Nursing,
77, 91
American Beverage Institute, 52
American Cancer Society, 13, 14, 15, 34, 40,
44
American Heart Association, 13, 14, 15, 34,
40, 44
American Legacy Foundation, 41
American Lung Association, 13, 14, 34, 40, 44
American Public Health Association, 119
Americans for Nonsmokers' Rights, 8
Anheuser-Busch, 65, 66
Annual Report (1972), 164–165

Annual Report (1973), 170, 171, 186
Annual Report (1974), 186–187, 189
Annual Report (1975), 173, 187
Annual Report (1976), 173
Annual Report (2001), 195
Arganbright, K., 60
Asian Pacific Partners for Empowerment and
Leadership, 41
ASSIST (American Stop Smoking Interven-
tion Study) [National Cancer Institute],
32, 38
The Atlas, 113–114, 121
Austin High School (Chicago), 133
Austin Violence Prevention Consortium, 132

B

Baird, J., 60–61
Barker, D., 120, 121
Beachler, M., 13, 31, 32, 39
Beck, J., 168
Bednash, G., 77, 82
Bekemeier, B., 119
Berkowitz, B., 104, 106, 117
Binge drinking: College Alcohol Study on,
53–54; definition of, 51; unappreciated
consequences of, 51–53
Bishop, J., 69
Blendon, R., 163–164, 167
B'nai Brith Hillel Foundation, 160
Bornemeier, J., 3, 4, 30
Boston CeaseFire Program, 136–138
Boston Police Department, 136
Boston Ten-Point Coalition, 137
Bowling for Columbine (movie), 129
Boys Scouts, 160
Bridging the Gap program, 8
Brodeur, P., 99, 100

Bruce, T., 102

Building Responsibility (University of Delaware), 69–70

C

California Proposition 99, 32

Campaign for Tobacco-Free Kids (the Center), 15

Carnegie Corporation of New York, 164, 166, 188

Casady, T., 57, 58

Case Western Reserve, 166

CDC (Centers for Disease Control and Prevention): College Alcohol Study influence on, 54; NAC partnership with, 41; RWJ's consultation with, 32; social marketing CD ROM based on work done by, 107; support for state work on tobacco prevention/treatment by, 37; on tobacco use by Americans, 6–7

CDC Health Alert Network funds, 110

CeaseFire Week (Chicago), 146

The Center. *See* National Center for Tobacco-Free Kids

Center on Alcohol Marketing and Youth, 56

The Center for Consumer Freedom, 52

Center for Health Administration Studies (University of Chicago), 167

Center for Health Care Strategies, 194

Center for Health and Health Care in Schools (George Washington University), 194

Center for the Health Professions (UCSF), 92–93

Center for Law and the Public's Health, 107

Center for Prevention Research (University of Kentucky), 194

Center for Tobacco Control Research and Education (UCSF), 22

Center for Tobacco-Free Kids, 41

CFP (call for proposals), 180–181, 187

Chaloupka, F., 12

Chicago: CeaseFire Week in, 146; violence/murder rates in, 129

Chicago Community Trust, 128, 134

Chicago Police Department, 129, 132, 133

Chicago Project Steering Committee, 134

Chicago Project for Violence Prevention: in the context of national gun violence,

146–147; eight-point plan used by, 134; funding of, 127–128; identifying infrastructure to implement, 131–133; inside workings of the, 138–140; lessons from Boston CeaseFire Program for, 136–138; Local Initiative Funding Partners Program funding of, 128, 134–136, 148; meeting the drug dealers, 143–145; neighborhood presence of workers from, 140–141; neighborhood return of outreach workers from, 141–143, 146; origins of, 127–128, 129–131; sharing the lessons learned from, 147–149

Chow, M., 93, 96

Christ Church of New Brunswick, 160

Clinical Nurse Scholars Program, 83–85

Clinical Scholars Program, 166–167, 168, 186, 188

Cluff, L., 84

Coalition for Tobacco-Free Colorado, 35–36

Collaborative on Performance Management, 111

Colleagues in Caring: Regional Collaboratives for Nursing Work Force Development, 90–92

College Alcohol Study (RWJ), 53–54, 55, 57

Committee for the Study of the Future of Public Health, 102

Commonwealth Fund, 164, 166, 167, 172, 188

Community Health Institute (New Hampshire), 109, 110

Community Hospital–Medical Staff Group Practices Program, 187

Connecticut Coalition to Stop Underage Drinking, 66

Controlling youth drinking programs: A Matter of Degree (LSU), 48–57, 62–67; Minnesota Join Together Coalition to Reduce Underage Drinking, 64–65; NU Directions (University of Nebraska–Lincoln), 52, 57–62; observations and recommendations on, 67–70; Reducing Underage Drinking Through Coalitions, 48, 54–56, 63–70; Texans Standing Tall, 65, 66. *See also* Youth drinking

Cornhusker Place, Inc. (Lincoln), 60

Covenant for Peace in Action, 138

Covington & Burling, 36
Curry, S., 22

D

Dahl, J., 119
Daley, R., 137
Davis, K., 167
DeJong, W., 54
Dental Training for Care of the Handicapped, 187
Department of Family Practice (UCD), 80
Diehl, D., 127, 128
Dixson, R., 159, 161
Doctors Ought to Care, 33
Domingue, C., 49, 62
Donaho, B., 86
Doyle, J., 52
Drinking. *See* Alcohol use; Youth drinking
Drug dealers, 143–145
Duke Medical School, 166

E

Educating Primary Care Practitioners in Their Home Communities: Partnerships for Training report, 90
Educational Testing Service, 171
Emmert, M., 49–50
EMS (Emergency Medical Services Program), 168, 187, 188–189, 193
Environmental Protection Agency, 117
Executive Nurse Fellows Program, 92–93

F

FDA (Food and Drug Administration): announces control over tobacco advertising/marketing by, 37; given authority to regulate tobacco (1997), 16–17; rule on nicotine regulation (1996) by, 12, 15
Federal Trade Commission, 21
Fighting Back, 6
Florida State University, 53
Ford, E., 184
Ford Foundation, 160, 162, 164, 167, 168, 184–186, 191
Ford, H., 184
Forrestal Center (Princeton University), 169
Foster, L., 162
Francis E. Parker Memorial Home (New Brunswick), 160
Frontier Nursing Service (Kentucky), 81

G

Gang turf violence, 143
Gardner, J. R., 155
George, F. Cardinal (Archbishop of Chicago), 137, 138
Gerlach, K. K., 29
Gimarc, D., 114
Girls Scouts, 160
Glantz, S., 22–23
Grande, D., 39
Griesen, J., 57

H

Haire, J., 65
Harden, B., 137
Hardiman, T., 143, 146
Harrison, A. R., 155
Harty, K., 39
Harvard School of Public Health College Alcohol Study (1993), 51
Harwood, E., 68
Hassmiller, S., 94–96, 117, 118, 121
Health Care's Human Crisis: The American Nursing Shortage study (RWJ, 2002)
Health Policy Fellows Program, 188
HEDIS (Health Plan Employer Data and Information Set), 19
Helene Fuld Health Trust, 77
Hill, L. F., 161
Hill-Burton Act (1948), 75
Holman, W., Jr., 161
Homicide rates: Chicago, 129; Chicago Project in context of gun violence and, 146–147. *See also* Chicago Project for Violence Prevention
Hospital Research & Education Foundation, 113
Houston, T., 33
Hughes, R. G., 7–8, 177

I

IDEO (California), 95
IHI (Institute for Healthcare Improvement), 95
I'M READY (University of Illinois at Chicago), 87
Independence Foundation, 77
Information Technology Collaborative, 106
Institute of Medicine (La Jolla), 102, 122

Irvin Foundation, 160

J

Jackson, R., 142, 143–145
Jacobson, P., 116
Jewish Healthcare Foundation, 77
John A. Hartford Foundation, 77
John D. and Catherine T. MacArthur Foundation, 127, 134, 135
Johns Hopkins Medical School, 166, 172
Johnson & Johnson, 155, 162, 186
Johnson, E., 158
Johnson, J., 157
Johnson, J. S., 158
Johnson, M., 157
Johnson New Brunswick Foundation, 158–160
Johnson, R. W.: early life of, 157; marriages of, 157–158; RWJ Foundation legacy of, 155–156
Johnson, R. W, II, 157
Johnson, R. W, III, 157–158
Johnson-Pawlson, J., 90
Join Together, 194
Jordan, J. T., 136
Joshiah Macy, Jr. Foundation, 77
Journal of the American Medical Association, 51
Journal of Public Health Management and Practice, 115

K

Kaiser Permanente, 93
Karel, F., 172, 173
Kassler, W., 109, 110
Kaufman, N., 9, 13, 14, 31, 102
Keenan, T., 79, 91, 92, 164, 167
Kellogg Foundation, 77, 100, 102, 104, 108, 114, 117–118, 122
Kennedy, D., 136
Kick Butts Day (the Center), 16
Koplan, J., 119
Koss, K., 52, 58–59

L

Lafronza, V., 118
Larkin, M. A., 29, 39
"Last Chance" shootings, 144
Lavizzo-Mourey, R., 24–25, 26, 43, 94
Leadership Development Collaborative, 106
Leadership to Keep Children Alcohol Free, 56

Levy, B., 119
The Lewin Group, 91–92, 93
L'Hommedieu, P., 161
Lienhard, G., 159, 161, 162, 163, 167, 173, 191
LINC (Ladders in Nursing Careers), 88–89
Linder, S., 116
Lobbying: NPO prohibitions regarding, 35–36; by tobacco industry, 33
Local Initiative Funding Partners Program, 128, 134–136, 148
LSU (Louisiana State University), decision to join A Matter of Degree by, 49–50, 52

M

MacArthur Foundation, 127, 134, 135
McCain, J., 17
McCoy, S., 142
McDermott, W., 163, 167
McGill Medical School, 166, 168
Macy, Jr. Foundation, 77
Mahoney, M., 164, 167
Major, L., 58
Managed care, 88
Martin, W. M., 161
Marx, J., 9
Master Settlement Agreement, 17
Mathews, N., 62
A Matter of Degree: goals and strategies used by, 56–57; grantmaking by, 56; LSU's experience with, 49–50, 52, 62–63; observations and recommendations on, 67–70; origins of, 54–56; programs funded by, 48; responses of students to, 52; University of Delaware's experience with, 69–70. *See also* RWJ (Robert Wood Johnson Foundation)
Maves, M., 43
Medicaid, 16, 183
Medicaid Managed Care Program, 194
Medicare, 183
Mendenhall Report, 167
Miami Herald, 172
Middlesex General Hospital, 157, 169
Mindus, D., 52
Minnesota Join Together Coalition to Reduce Underage Drinking, 64–65
Minors in Possession citation (NU Directions), 60

Monitoring the Future study (University of Michigan), 7
Mothers Against Drunk Driving, 47–48
Myers, M., 14, 15, 16, 17

N

NAC (National Advisory Committee): changing role of, 41; membership changes in, 40–41; restructuring of, 39; selection of program sites made by, 181
NACCHO (National Association of County and City Health Officials) [Washington, D.C.], 104, 118
Nachbar, J., 64
Najarian, G., 66
National Academy of Sciences, 169
National Academy of Sciences' Institute of Medicine report (1988), 102
National Action Network (the Center), 15–16
National Cancer Institute, 172
National Cancer Institute ASSIST, 32, 38
National Center for Tobacco-Free Kids: criticism of tobacco strategy by, 22–23; establishment of, 15; four goals and campaign by, 15–16, 17
National Committee on Quality Assurance, 19
National Excellence Collaboratives (Turning Point initiative): Nebraska implementation of, 108–109; New Hampshire implementation of, 109–110; New York State implementation of, 110–112; organization of, 106–107; South Carolina implementation of, 114–115; Virginia implementation of, 112–114
National Institute on Alcohol Abuse and Alcoholism, 54, 56
National Institutes of Health, 41, 183
National Planning Association, 171
National Spit Tobacco Education Program, tobacco-control strategy of, 8
National Tobacco Policy Initiative, 39
Nebraska Turning Point Project, 108–109
New Brunswick YMCA and YWCA, 160
New Hampshire Turning Point initiative, 109–110
New York coalition, 42
New York State Community Health Partnership, 111, 112
New York State Department of Health, 112

New York State Turning Point initiative, 110–112
New York Times, 162
New York Times Magazine, 168
Newbergh, C., 73
North Central Community Care Partnership, 108
North Country Health Consortium, 110
Northern New Hampshire Area Health Education Center, 110
Novelli, W. D., 15, 16
NPOs (National Program Offices): advantages/disadvantages of using external, 192t; announced closing of, 43; assessment of makeup of, 39; communication functions of, 182, 188–189; early assessment of approach used by, 189–193; evolution of, 193–196; formal program evaluations by, 181–182; lobbying prohibitions by, 35–36; during period between 1973–2002, 195t; potential of model of, 169; reflections on contributions of, 44–46; as RWJ grant-making mechanism, 179–180; selection of, 33; site visits/technical assistance provided by, 41–42, 44; six basic characteristics of, 180–182; state coalition grantees selected by, 34–35; variation among different, 194–196. *See also* RWJ (Robert Wood Johnson Foundation) grants
NU Directions (University of Nebraska–Lincoln): college social environment and, 58–59; education and information provided by, 60–61; evaluating achievements of, 61–62; neighborhood relations with, 59; on-campus policy and enforcement policies and, 59–60; origins of, 52, 57–58
Nurse Faculty Fellowships in Primary Care, 82, 84, 96
Nurse practitioner projects, 80–81
Nurse Recruitment Coalition (Pittsburgh), 87
Nursing education programs: Clinical Nurse Scholars, 83–85; Colleagues in Caring collaboratives for, 90–92; early accreditation/standards of, 75; early nurse practitioner, 79–82; Executive Nurse Fellows Program, 92–93; LINC (Ladders in Nursing Careers), 88–89; national programs for, 78fig; Nurse Faculty Fellowships in Primary Care, 82, 84, 96; Nursing Services

Nursing education programs *(continued)*
Manpower Development, 87; Partnerships for Training, 89–90; Strengthening Hospital Nursing, 85–87; Teaching Nursing Home, 82–83; Transformation of Care at the Bedside, 93–96

Nursing profession: reviewing RWJ's initiatives on, 96–97; RWJ support of the, 77, 79

Nursing Services Manpower Development Program, 87

Nursing shortage: addressed by Strengthening Hospital Nursing program, 85–87; current status of, 76–77; origins and development of, 75–76; as U.S. crisis, 75

O

Operation CeaseFire (Boston), 136–138
Or Forfeit Freedom (Johnson), 158
Oregon coalition, 42–43
Orleans, C. T., 1, 17

P

Palm, D., 108–109
Parker, S. G., 47, 48
Parks and Wildlife Foundation of Texas, 65
Partnership for a Drug-Free America, 6
Partnerships for Training, 89–90
Pearson, D., 158
Perez, F., 139–141, 143–145
Performance Management Collaborative, 107
Perry, S., 83–84, 85
Pertschuk, M., 21, 26
Pew Charitable Trusts, 56, 85
Pickett, A., 142–143
Pirani, S., 112
Porter Novelli, 15
Price, D. K., 168
Program to Equip Emergency Nurses with Primary Care Skills, 81, 82
Proposition 99 (California), 32
Public Health Statute Modernization Collaborative, 107

R

RAND Corporation, 171
Rapid Response strategies, 138
Rapson, M., 91, 92
Reducing Underage Drinking Through Coalitions: achievements of, 48; Connecticut Coalition, 66; early assessment of results by, 66–67; goals/objectives of, 63–64; Minnesota Join Together Coalition, 64–65; observations and recommendations on, 67–70; origins of, 54–56; RWJ requirements for, 63; Texans Standing Tall, 65–66; variety of approaches used by, 64–66

Regionalized Perinatal Care Program, 187
Remove Intoxicated Drivers, 47
Report of the Study for the Ford Foundation on Policy and Program, 184
Research Network on the Etiology of Tobacco Dependence, 194
Rivers, Rev. E., 137
Robbins, E., 36
Robert Wood Johnson University Hospital, 157
Rockefeller Foundation, 183
Rogers, D. E., 163, 164–165, 167, 169, 170–171, 172, 189, 190
Rogers, T., 120, 121, 156
Rosenfeld, R., 146–147
Ross, E. D., 157
RWJ *Annual Report* (1972), 164–165
RWJ *Annual Report* (1973), 170, 171, 186
RWJ *Annual Report* (1974), 186–187, 189
RWJ *Annual Report* (1975), 173, 187
RWJ *Annual Report* (1976), 173
RWJ *Annual Report* (2001), 195
RWJ (Robert Wood Johnson Foundation): criticism of strategy taken by, 22–23; cultural differences between Kellogg and, 117–118; establishment of, 155–156; IRS questioning of tax-exempt status of, 36; new direction taken by president of, 24–26; philosophy, programs, and people (1972–1975) of, 161–162, 162–173; reviewing tobacco strategy used by, 20–24; substance abuse mission undertaken by, 5–6, 7–9; summary of first four years of, 173; support of nursing profession by, 77, 79–97; tax issues affecting, 161, 162, 164, 186; tobacco-control research undertaken by, 9, 12–13; transition from local to national philanthropy (1968–1971), 160–162. *See also* A Matter of Degree

RWJ (Robert Wood Johnson Foundation) grants: comprehensive strategies for, 3–4;

critical decisions affecting approach of, 161–162; establishing system for making, 167–170; Ford Foundation experience influencing, 184–186; integrating evaluation and communications regarding, 170–173; tax issues affecting, 161, 162, 164, 186; treatment and cessation programs given, 17–20. *See also* NPOs (National Program Offices)

S

Sadler, B., 169
St. Peter's Hospital, 169
Santayana, G., 156
SAPRP (Substance Abuse Policy Research Program), 12, 13
Schneider Institute for Health Policy (Brandeis University), 19
School Health Service Program, 81, 82
Schroeder, S.: interest in substance abuse issue by, 5, 6; partnership with AMA suggested by, 13; regarding RWJ's tobacco-control work, 20–21; research strategy directed by, 9; support of programs to reduce youth drinking by, 53; tobacco-control agenda of, 31
Scientific American, 146
Scrimshaw, S., 130
Seitz, P., 135–136, 148
September 11th attacks, 117, 119
Shapiro, S., 138–139
Sidel, V., 119
Slade, J., 12
Slutkin, G., 128, 129–132, 137–138, 140, 147, 148–149
Smaller War Plants Corporation, 158
Smith, G., 102
Smoke in Their Eyes: Lessons in Movement Leadership from the Tobacco Wars (Pertschuk), 21
Smoke-Free Families, 8, 13–14, 29–30
SmokeLess States program: achievements of individual state coalitions in, 42–43; early challenges faced by, 34–36; establishment and development of, 31–34; establishment of, 13; evolution of the, 37–38; reflections and recommendations on, 43–46; renewal of focus on tobacco policy by, 38–43

Social Marketing National Excellence Collaborative, 107, 111
Society of St. Vincent de Paul (Highland Park), 169
Socolar, R., 115, 116
South Carolina Turning Point initiative, 114–115
Stanford Medical School, 166
STAT (Stop Teenage Addiction to Tobacco), 6
Statewide Tobacco Prevention and Control, 39
Stewart, J., 110
Strengthening Hospital Nursing, 85–87
Students Against Drunk Driving, 47
Substance abuse: RWJ Foundation's combating of, 5–6; scourge of, 5. *See also* Tobacco use; Youth drinking
Substance Abuse Policy Research Program, 21
SUNY (State University of New York), 111
Surgeon General's report, 7, 20

T

T2B2 (Third Thursday Breakfast Broadcasts), 112
Tax Reform Act (1969), 161, 162, 164, 186
Teaching Nursing Home Program, 82–83
Texans Standing Tall program, 65, 66
Texas Parks & Wildlife Department, 65
Texas Parks & Wildlife magazine, 66
Thomas, E., 59
Thompson, D., 161
Tobacco advertising: FDA announces control over, 37; Reducing Underage Drinking coalitions efforts to control, 65
Tobacco cessation/treatment programs: reduced emphasis by RWJ on, 24–26; RWJ grants given to, 17–20
Tobacco industry: lobbying by, 33; state lawsuits against, 38–39
Tobacco Institute, 14–15
Tobacco in Managed Care (RWJ), 19
Tobacco Policy Research and Evaluation Program, 21, 31, 37
Tobacco research: RWJ's entrance into, 9, 12–13; Tobacco Institute's efforts to fend off, 14–15
Tobacco use: CDC statistics on, 6–7; Surgeon General's report on, 7. *See also* Substance abuse
Tobacco-control grants, 10*t*–11*t*

Tobacco-Control Section (California Department of Health Services), 41

TPREP (Tobacco Policy Research and Evaluation Program) [RWJ], formation of, 9, 12

Transformation of Care at the Bedside, 93–96

Turning Point initiative: use of bioterrorism funds for, 119–120; conceptual bases of, 115–117; controversies and issues of, 115–120; implementation phase of, 107–115, 117–118; introduction to, 99–100; National Excellence Collaborative to implement, 106–115; origins of, 102–104; planning phase of, 105; public health issues focused on by, 120–121

Turning Point initiative implementation: controversies and issues during, 117–118; in Nebraska, 108–109; in New Hampshire, 109–110; in New York State, 110–112; in South Carolina, 114–115; in Virginia, 112–114

Turning Point Model State Public Health Act, 107

Turning Point National Advisory Committee, 104

Turning Point National Program Office (Seattle), 104

"TurningPointSpeak," 116

Tuskegee Institute (Alabama), 80–81

U

Underage drinking. *See* Youth drinking

United Community Services of Central Jersey, 169

University of Colorado at Boulder, 52

University of Delaware Building Responsibility program, 69–70

University of Nebraska–Lincoln's NU Directions, 52, 57–62

Utah Valley Hospital (Provo), 80

V

Violence: Chicago murder rates and, 129; Chicago Project in context of national gun, 146–147; gang turf, 143. *See also* Chicago Project for Violence Prevention

Virginia Atlas of Community Health, 113–114, 121

Virginia Center for Healthy Communities, 113

Virginia Hospital & Healthcare Association, 113

Virginia Hospital Research & Education Foundation, 112–113

Virginia Turning Point initiative, 112–114

Viser, P., 90

Vrzal, M., 61–62

W

Waddell, L., 114, 115

Wall Street Journal, 16

Walter D. Matheny School, 160

Ward, E., 66

Warner, K., 12, 25–26

Warren, F., 89–90

Washington Post, 137

Web sites: on the Center and tobacco control information, 16; by NU Directions local events, 58

Wechsler, H., 53, 54, 62–63

Weitzman, E., 63, 69

Wentz, S., 36

Wilson, J., 113–114

W.K. Kellogg Foundation, 77, 100, 102, 104, 108, 114, 117–118, 122

Wood, J. W., 36

Woodruff Health Sciences Center (Emory University), 119

Workman, T., 61

World Conference on Tobacco OR Health (1994), 14

World Health Organization, 129

World Report on Violence and Health, 129

Wynne, B., 62

Y

Yardley, O., 60

Yoast, R., 68, 70

Youth Advocates of the Year Awards (the Center), 16

Youth drinking: binge, 51; consequences of, 50–51; raising public consciousness about, 47–48; as serious health problem, 47. *See also* Alcohol use; Controlling youth drinking programs; Substance abuse

⎯ᴍ⎯Table of Contents
To Improve Health and Health Care 1997

Foreword
Steven A. Schroeder

Introduction
Stephen L. Isaacs and James R. Knickman

Acknowledgments

1 **Reach Out: Physicians' Initiative to Expand Care to Underserved Americans**
Irene M. Wielawski

2 **Improving the Health Care Workforce: Perspectives from Twenty-Four Years' Experience**
Stephen L. Isaacs, Lewis G. Sandy, and Steven A. Schroeder

3 **A Review of the National Access-to-Care Surveys**
Marc L. Berk and Claudia L. Schur

4 **Expertise Meets Politics: Efforts to Work with States**
Beth A. Stevens and Lawrence D. Brown

5 **The Media and Change in Health Systems**
Marc S. Kaplan and Mark A. Goldberg

6 **Addressing the Problem of Medical Malpractice**
Joel C. Cantor, Robert A. Berenson, Julia S. Howard, and Walter Wadlington

7 **Unmet Need in the Community: The Springfield Study**
Susan M. Allen and Vincent Mor

8 **Unexpected Returns: Insights from SUPPORT**
Joanne Lynn

9 **Developing Child Immunization Registries: The All Kids Count Program**
Gordon H. DeFriese, Kathleen M. Faherty, Victoria A. Freeman, Priscilla A. Guild, Delores A. Musselman, William C. Watson, Jr., and Kristin Nicholson Saarlas

10 **The Homeless Families Program: A Summary of Key Findings**
Debra J. Rog and Marjorie Gutman

11 **The National Health and Social Life Survey: Public Health Findings and Their Implications**
Robert T. Michael

–w–Table of Contents

To Improve Health and Health Care 1998–1999

Foreword
Steven A. Schroeder
Introduction
Stephen L. Isaacs and James R. Knickman
Acknowledgments

Combating Substance Abuse

1 Adopting the Substance Abuse Goal: A Story of Philanthropic Decision Making
Robert G. Hughes

2 Tobacco Policy Research
Marjorie A. Gutman, David G. Altman, and Robert L. Rabin

3 The National Spit Tobacco Education Program
Leonard Koppett

4 Alcohol and Work: Results from a Corporate Drinking Study
Thomas W. Mangione, Jonathan Howland, and Marianne Lee

Increasing Access to Care

5 Influencing Academic Health Centers:
The Robert Wood Johnson Foundation Experience
Lewis G. Sandy and Richard Reynolds

6 The Strengthening Hospital Nursing Program
Thomas G. Rundall, David B. Starkweather, and Barbara Norrish

Improving Chronic Care

7 Faith in Action
Paul Jellinek, Terri Gibbs Appel, and Terrance Keenan

8 Providing Care—Not Cure—for Patients with Chronic Conditions
Lisa Lopez

9 The Mental Health Services Program for Youth
Leonard Saxe and Theodore P. Cross

Communications

10 The Foundation's Radio and Television Grants, 1987–1997
Victoria D. Weisfeld

A Look Back

11 Support of Nurse Practitioners and Physician Assistants
Terrance Keenan

—ᴡ—Table of Contents
To Improve Health and Health Care 2000

Foreword
Steven A. Schroeder
Introduction
Stephen L. Isaacs and James R. Knickman
Acknowledgments

Access to Care

1 **School-Based Health Clinics**
   Paul Brodeur

2 **Expanding Health Insurance for Children**
   Marguerite Y. Holloway

3 **The Minority Medical Education Program**
   Lois Bergeisen and Joel C. Cantor

Services for People with Chronic Conditions

4 **Coming Home: Affordable Assisted Living for the Rural Elderly**
   Joseph Alper

5 **Adult Day Centers**
   Rona Smyth Henry, Nancy J. Cox, Burton V. Reifler, and Carolyn Asbury

6 **The Program on Chronic Mental Illness**
   Howard H. Goldman

Research

7 **Research as a Foundation Strategy**
   James R. Knickman

8 **Linking Biomedical and Behavioral Research
   for Tobacco Use Prevention: Sundance and Beyond**
   Nancy J. Kaufman and Karyn L. Feiden

Collaboration with Other Philanthropies

9 **The Local Initiative Funding Partners Program**
   Irene M. Wielawski

A Look Back

10 **The Emergency Medical Services Program**
   Digby Diehl

Appendix

Twenty-Five Years of Emergency Medical Systems: A Retrospective
James C. Butler and Susan G. Fowler

~ɯ~Table of Contents

To Improve Health and Health Care 2001

Foreword
Steven A. Schroeder

Editors' Introduction: Grantmaking Insights from The Robert Wood Johnson Foundation *Anthology*
Stephen L. Isaacs and James R. Knickman

Acknowledgments

Inside the Foundation

1 Expanding the Focus of The Robert Wood Johnson Foundation: Health as an Equal Partner to Health Care
J. Michael McGinnis and Steven A. Schroeder

2 "Getting the Word Out": A Foundation Memoir and Personal Journey
Frank Karel

Programs

3 Children's Health Initiatives
Sharon Begley and Ruby P. Hearn

4 The Changing Approach to Managed Care77
Janet Firshein and Lewis G. Sandy

5 Integrating Acute and Long-Term Care for the Elderly
Joseph Alper and Rosemary Gibson

6 The Workers' Compensation Health Initiative: At the Convergence of Work and Health
Allard E. Dembe and Jay S. Himmelstein

7 Sound Partners for Community Health
Digby Diehl

A Look Back

8 The Regionalized Perinatal Care Program
Marguerite Y. Holloway

9 Improving Dental Care
Paul Brodeur

Collaboration with Other Philanthropies

10 Partnership Among National Foundations: Between Rhetoric and Reality
Stephen L. Isaacs and John H. Rodgers

—ɯ—Table of Contents

To Improve Health and Health Care Volume V

Foreword
Steven A. Schroeder

Editors' Introduction: Strategies for Improving Access to Health Care—Observations from The Robert Wood Johnson Foundation *Anthology* Series
Stephen L. Isaacs and James R. Knickman

Acknowledgments

Programs

1 The Nurse Home Visitation Program
Joseph Alper

2 Tuberculosis: Old Disease, New Challenge
Carolyn Newbergh

3 Programs to Improve the Health of Native Americans
Paul Brodeur

4 Service Credit Banking
Susan Dentzer

5 Consumer Choice in Long-term Care
A. E. Benjamin and Rani E. Snyder

6 The Health Policy Fellowships Program
Richard S. Frank

A Closer Look

7 Recovery High School
Digby Diehl

8 *On Doctoring*: The Making of an Anthology of Literature and Medicine
Richard C. Reynolds and John Stone

A Look Back

9 The Foundation and AIDS: Behind the Curve but Leading the Way
Ethan Bronner

Inside the Foundation

10 Program-Related Investments
Marco Navarro and Peter Goodwin

11 Tending Our Backyard: The Robert Wood Johnson Foundation's Grantmaking in New Jersey
Pamela S. Dickson

~ᴍ~Table of Contents

To Improve Health and Health Care Volume VI

Foreword
Steven A. Schroeder

Editors' Introduction
Stephen L. Isaacs and James R. Knickman

Acknowledgments

Section One: Reflections on Health, Philanthropy, and The Robert Wood Johnson Foundation

  1 A Conversation with Steven A. Schroeder
     Renie Schapiro

Section Two: Improving Health Care

  2 The Health Tracking Initiative
     Carolyn Newbergh

  3 Practice Sights: State Primary Care Development Strategies
     Irene M. Wielawski

  4 The Foundation's End-of-Life Programs:
     Changing the American Way of Death
     Ethan Bronner

Section Three: Improving Health

  5 The Center for Tobacco-Free Kids and
     the Tobacco-Settlement Negotiations
     Digby Diehl

  6 Helping Addicted Smokers Quit: The Foundation's
     Tobacco-Cessation Programs
     C. Tracy Orleans and Joseph Alper

  7 Combating Alcohol Abuse in Northwestern New Mexico:
     Gallup's Fighting Back and Healthy Nations Programs
     Paul Brodeur

Section Four: Strengthening Human Capacity

  8 Building Health Policy Research Capacity in the Social Sciences
     David C. Colby

  9 The Robert Wood Johnson Community Health Leadership Program
     Paul Mantell

Section Five: Communications

  10 The Covering Kids Communications Campaign
     Susan B. Garland

Section Six: A Look Back

  11 The Swing-Bed Program
     Sharon Begley

—ₘ—Table of Contents

To Improve Health and Health Care Volume VII

Foreword
Risa Lavizzo-Mourey

Editors' Introduction: Observations on Grantmaking from
The Robert Wood Johnson Foundation *Anthology* Series
Stephen L. Isaacs and James R. Knickman

Acknowledgments

Section One: Targeted Portfolio

1 The Fighting Back Program
Irene M. Wielawski

2 Join Together and CADCA: Backing Up the Front Line
Paul Jellinek and Renie Schapiro

3 The Robert Wood Johnson Foundation's Efforts
to Contain Health Care Costs
Carolyn Newbergh

4 The Teaching Nursing Home Program
Ethan Bronner

Section Two: Human Capital Portfolio

5 The Robert Wood Johnson Clinical Scholars
Program
*Jonathan Showstack, Arlyss Anderson Rothman,
Laura C. Leviton, and Lewis G. Sandy*

6 The Robert Wood Johnson Foundation's Commitment
to Increasing Minorities in the Health Professions
Jane Isaacs Lowe and Constance M. Pechura

7 The National Health Policy Forum
Richard S. Frank

Section Three: Vulnerable Populations Portfolio

8 The Injury Free Coalition for Kids
Paul Brodeur

9 The Homeless Prenatal Program
Digby Diehl

Section Four: Pioneering Portfolio

10 The Robert Wood Johnson Foundation's
Response to Emergencies: September 11th,
Bioterrorism, and Natural Disasters
Stephen L. Isaacs